MW01502609

VITREOUS SUBSTITUTES

VITREOUS
SUBSTITUTES

Gholam A. Peyman, MD
Professor of Ophthalmology
Chief of Vitreoretinal Surgery
Louisiana State University Eye Center
New Orleans, Louisiana

Joel A. Schulman, MD
Associate Professor of Ophthalmology
Louisiana State University Medical Center
Shreveport, Louisiana

APPLETON & LANGE
East Norwalk, Connecticut

Copyright © 1995 by Appleton & Lange
A Simon & Schuster Company

95 96 97 98 99 / 10 9 8 7 6 5 4 3 2 1

Prentice Hall International (UK) Limited, *London*
Prentice Hall of Australia Pty. Limited, *Sydney*
Prentice Hall Canada, Inc., *Toronto*
Prentice Hall Hispanoamericana, S.A., *Mexico*
Prenctice Hall of India Private Limited, *New Delhi*
Prentice Hall of Japan, Inc., *Tokyo*
Simon and Schuster Asia Pte. Ltd., *Singapore*
Editora Prentice Hall do Brasil Ltda., *Rio de Janeiro*
Prentice Hall, *Englewood Cliffs, New Jersey*

Library of Congress Cataloging-in-Publication Data

Peyman, Gholam A., 1935-
    Vitreous substitutes / Gholam A. Peyman, Joel A. Schulman.
        p. cm.
    Includes bibliographical references and index.
    ISBN 0-8385-9484-0
    1. Vitreous substitutes. I. Schulman, Joel A.
    [DNLM: 1. Vitrectomy—methods. 2. Retinal Detachment—surgery.
    3. Implants, Artificial. 4. Silicone Oils. 5. Fluorocarbons.
    6. Gases. WW 250 P515v 1995]
    RE992.V57P49 1995
    617.7´4—dc20
    DNLM/DLC   94-39562
    for Library of Congress   CIP

Acquisitions Editor: Jane Licht
Production Editor: Elizabeth Ryan
Designer: Mary Skudlarek
Production Service: Ruttle, Shaw, & Wetherill, Inc.

ISBN 0-8385-9484-0

90000

9 780838 594841

PRINTED IN THE UNITED STATES OF AMERICA

Contents

CHAPTER 3. PERFLUOROCARBON LIQUIDS

Preface

In the daily practice of any medical specialty, physicians walk the halls of the history of all the work that has gone before. Whether we stop to reflect on the past or not, we owe the present, in part, to the notable achievements of pioneers in our respective fields. This tradition of building on the past can be traced to the earliest days of medicine. Hippocrates, four centuries before Christ, wrote in his *Aphorisms,* "Life is short, art long, opportunity fleeting, experience treacherous, judgment difficult." We now call Hippocrates the "father of medicine," and he is rightly credited with laying the foundations of scientific medicine. Nevertheless, one can deduce from his words that he must have realized his own work was just a beginning, a foundation upon which others would build.

In ophthalmology, we too can gain a useful perspective on the state of the art of our own field by recalling earlier works. In the last three decades, progress in vitreoretinal surgery has moved hand in hand with the development of vitreous substitutes such as silicone oil, long-acting gases, and perfluorocarbon liquids (PFCLs).

Two pioneers in this field have been largely overlooked, and so we have featured them in this book: Dr. Paul Cibis and Dr. Leland Clark. Dr. Cibis pioneered the use of silicone oil in ophthalmology, but he died young and never received the credit he deserved. In fact, his approach was strongly criticized in the United States at the time. Dr. Clark introduced PFCLs in ophthalmology, but his contribution and his work are largely unrecognized to this day.

SILICONE OIL

In the early 1960s, Cibis and Stone and other investigators implanted silicone oil in the vitreous of animals and in humans for the first time to provide a permanent support for the detached retina. But it took three decades, as well as a great deal of courage and perseverance by numerous investigators (Scott, Živojnović, Leaver, Labelle, Lean), to fully convert the ophthalmic community to its use. Now, silicone oil has become an indispensable tool in the management of complex cases of retinal surgery.

LONG-ACTING GASES

Although air was used by Ohm to tamponade the detached retina over 80 years ago, clinical applications of long-acting gases first appeared in the early 1970s. Initiated by Lincoff, Norton, and researchers in our laboratory, the advent of long-acting gases represented a major breakthrough in terms of wide clinical applications. Recently, Hilton, Dominguez, Grizzard, and Tornambe popularized the use of gases for pneumatic retinopexy in uncomplicated retinal detachment. This office procedure simplified treatment of routine cases in retinal detachment, and it has become the standard of care in outpatient surgery.

PERFLUOROCARBON LIQUIDS

PFCLs were developed by Clark in the 1960s as oxygen carriers and blood substitutes. It was ironically serendipitous that Clark suffered a retinal detachment himself. This personal misfortune motivated him to introduce PFCLs as a heavier-than-water substance to ophthalmology, where they could be used in reattaching the retina.

Haidt, Zimmerman, Miyamoto, Chang, and our group contributed to the further development of PFCLs. In contrast to other vitreous substitutes, PFCLs have been eagerly embraced by vitreoretinal surgeons because their development was concurrent with other modern vitreoretinal surgical techniques. PFCLs have now become an indispensable part of management of giant retinal tears, dislocated lenses, and proliferative vitreoretinopathy. PFCLs have contributed significantly to increased success rates of these complex cases.

This book provides a timely update of the works of numerous investigators and clinicians in this still evolving field. It gathers together up-to-date information on silicone oil, gases, and PFCLs, including detailed descriptions of surgical techniques used with their applications. The book can also serve as a review for those interested in vitreoretinal surgery.

On a personal note of acknowledgment, we are in debt to—and we sincerely thank—the many individuals who have helped us in this endeavor: co-workers, colleagues, fellows and students, and friends. Without them and their continuous support, this work would not have been possible.

Special thanks are due to Ms. Mary Winnike, librarian at the Department of Ophthalmology, University of Illinois at Chicago, for reviewing the references. We are especially in debt to Ms. Trisha Chiasson and Mr. Pat Adkins for their fine editorial assistance. Ms. Linda Warren beautified the book with her artistic drawings and illustrations. Finally, we thank our publisher's editor, Ms. Jane Licht, for her help and cooperation.

Gholam A. Peyman, MD
Joel A. Schulman, MD

Paul Anton Cibis, MD

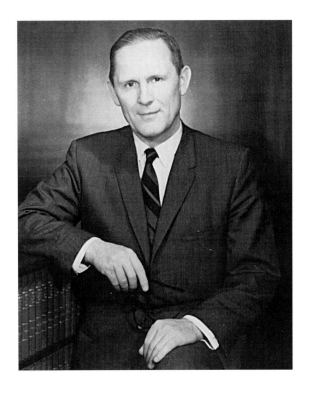

More than any other individual, Paul Cibis may be credited with the introduction and popularization of intravitreal surgery. Born in Silesia in 1911, he was educated in medicine in Breslau, Munich, Berlin, and Heidelberg. His interest in eye surgery grew out of the two years he spent on the Russian front during World War II and the three years he was Oberartzt at the University of Heidelberg, which served as a military hospital. He was awarded the Graefe prize by the German Ophthalmologic Society in 1949 for work on local adaptation of the retina, and emigrated to the United States that same year. He became a research ophthalmologist for the American Air Force, first at the School of Aerospace Medicine, Randolph Field, San Antonio, Texas, and later at Washington University in St. Louis, where he served as an associate professor until his untimely death in 1965.

A multifaceted scientist, Dr. Cibis developed several surgical devices, including sutures, implants, and sheets for use in orbit floor repair. Goldmann considered his theory of color vision to be his most important contribution. In 1954 he coauthored a paper on the histology of retinal burns in rabbits exposed to atomic blasts, suggesting that high-intensity light might be used therapeutically to coagulate the retina. When photocoagulation was introduced two years later, he became one of the first surgeons in the United States to use that therapy.

Dr. Cibis's interest in the surgical treatment of retinal detachments led to his study of the vitreous. That, in turn, led to his ground-breaking use of silicone oil as a vitreous substitute. Despite early setbacks, opposition, and criticism, he never lost faith in his work.

Leland C. Clark, Jr., PhD

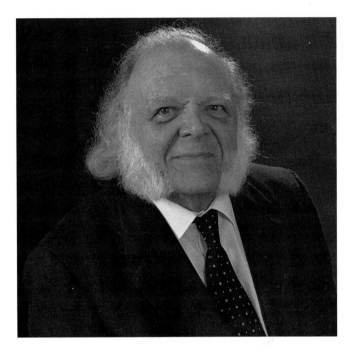

In addition to his ground-breaking work with fluorocarbon liquids, Dr. Clark has contributed to many different areas of science in medicine and ophthalmology. After graduating with honors from Antioch College in 1941 with a Bachelor of Science degree in chemistry, he performed postgraduate work at the University of Rochester College of Medicine and Dentistry under a National Research Council Fellowship. Receiving his PhD in 1944, he returned to the Antioch campus in Yellow Springs, Ohio, where he established a biochemistry department in the Fels Research Institute. While studying vitamin, enzyme, and steroid metabolism in normal children, he began work on a machine capable of performing the functions of the heart and lungs. In 1949 he built a prototype that adequately supplied oxygen to a dog; this research led to a collaboration with the Children's Hospital Research Foundation in Cincinnati, where the heart-lung machine was further perfected and many techniques of open-heart surgery were developed.

Recognizing the usefulness of measuring oxygen tension in blood quickly, both during and after heart surgery, Dr. Clark invented the Clark Electrode in 1954, an oxygen sensor that led to the development of many other on-the-spot instruments for intensive care use.

In 1958, Dr. Clark set up an open-heart surgery unit in the Department of Surgery in Birmingham, Alabama. He developed new, rapid methods to measure blood levels of glucose, lactate, alcohol, and cholesterol and methods of continuously recording the availability of oxygen in the brains of live animals. His concept of enzymes combined with electrodes started the now flourishing biosensor technology field. In 1992 he was honored for this work with an award at the International Biosensor Conference in Geneva, Switzerland.

Dr. Clark's interest in ophthalmology began as a result of suffering from a retinal detachment in 1980. This led to the development of perfluorocarbon liquid as a heavier-than-water substance to tamponade and reattach the retina.

Dr. Clark is presently Research Professor of Biological Sciences at Antioch College. There he is continuing his work for eye surgery, fluorocarbons for breathing, artificial blood, angioplasty, and biosensors. He received the medical school's highest honor, the Drake award, in June 1993. Currently he is Vice President of Research and Development and a director of Synthetic Blood International, Inc.

Chapter 1
Silicone Oil

SILICONE OILS

Silicone oil (polydimethylsiloxane, or PDMS) is a term used to designate any of the viscous hydrophobic polymer compounds based on siloxane chemistry. Regardless of the exact chemistry, all silicone oils share SiO units. The length of the polymer determines the viscosity of a silicone oil. The longer the polymer, the greater the viscosity. When two different polydimethylsiloxanes with different polymer lengths are mixed, a silicone oil of intermediate viscosity results.[1,2]

The silicone oils most commonly used as vitreous substitutes in the treatment of complicated retinal detachments are the polydimethylsiloxanes. Unless otherwise stated, all references to silicone oil refer to these substances.[3]

Polydimethylsiloxane (Fig. 1–1) is produced by the polymerization of oligodimethyl siloxane molecules [-(CH3)$_2$ SiO].[2,4] The resulting chemical process produces a PDMS containing a large number of molecules of a mean molecular weight but also including some low-molecular-weight molecules (LMW) and an even smaller number of slightly higher-molecular-weight molecules. High-viscosity silicone oils have reduced amounts of low-molecular-weight components (LMWCs) compared with lower-viscosity oils.[2,5,6]

Molecular weight distribution of PDMS can be measured by gel permeation chromatography or by testing for volatility. Testing for volatility involves keeping the PDMS for 24 hours at 200°C and then determining weight loss. The LMWCs are more volatile.[2,5]

The LMWCs consist of small, ring-shaped cyclosiloxanes (300 to 800 MW) and slightly larger linear molecules (800 to 2,400 MW), both of which are highly volatile. As a result, LMWCs are able to diffuse as a vapor into adjacent tissue and possibly cause inflammatory toxic reaction or macrophage migration. The diffusion of LMWCs into different tissue can be followed by their condensation into droplets. The temperature gradient, with a cooler temperature in the anterior than in the posterior segment of the eye, favors condensation in the anterior chamber.[2,5]

Catalyst remnants are another component of polymerization. Despite being inactivated during the polymerization procedure, these catalysts still may react toxically with neighboring tissue, causing significant adverse effects.[2,5,7]

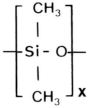

Figure 1–1. Chemical composition of dimethylsiloxane.

To provide better biocompatibility, the chemical purity of silicone oil is important. The number of LMWCs should be restricted. The silicone oil also needs to be purified to eliminate catalysts with an electric resistivity not less than 10^{14} Ω.[2,5,7]

Silicone, an inert, transparent substance, has a refractive index of 1.4035, which is slightly higher than that of vitreous. The viscosity of the fluid used intraocularly varies from 1,000 to 12,500 cSt. Unlike most other vitreous substitutes, silicone may remain in the eye almost permanently.[8]

Silicone fluids are nonwettable, moisture repellent, and impermeable to solutes but allow diffusion of gases and water vapor. Those with viscosities greater than 50 cSt are heat stable and thus may be sterilized with heat.[9]

The silicone–water interfacial tension (40 dyne/cm^2) is high, but still less than that of the gas–water interface (70 dyne/cm^2). Surface tension is not affected by viscosity. Because its density is 0.975, 3% less than water, silicone oil floats on water in the vitreous. Regardless of position, silicone oil is always found at the top of the vitreous cavity. It is impossible to fill the vitreous cavity completely with silicone because of the pressure exerted by a small amount of intraocular fluid located between the bottom of the bubble and the retina. Superior tears are always closed by the silicone oil bubble, but inferior tears frequently require a scleral buckle to achieve permanent closure.

Because the refractive index of silicone is close to that of water, surgical maneuvers under silicone oil are easily visible. This facilitates postoperative examination of the retina and allows early postoperative visual rehabilitation in eyes with good visual potential. Compared with gas, silicone oil provides a longer-term internal tamponade, which is important when an initially closed retinal break is expected to reopen. Reopening can occur in eyes with proliferative vitreoretinopathy (PVR) after a gas tamponade has been reabsorbed; in such cases, the break edge may rise because of retinal shortening around breaks. Besides providing continued closure of the break while remaining inside the eye as a tamponading agent, silicone oil also prevents subretinal fluid from accumulating through the break, which could result in a retinal detachment.

An air–fluid interface has a higher surface tension than does a fluid–silicone boundary. Air–fluid exchange may be used initially to flatten the retina; then the air may be replaced with silicone oil to provide a long-term internal tamponade.[10-14]

Silicone oil has a higher refractive index than vitreous (1.33); for this reason, injection of silicone oil into the vitreous cavity results in a notable change in the refractive index of the eye.

Smith et al[15] examined refractive changes in 34 silicone-filled eyes. Because the refractive index of silicone oil is higher than that of aqueous or lens cortex, the change in refractive error is determined by the shape of the anterior refractive surface of the silicone bubble. A negative lens was found in phakic eyes in which the oil surface is concave because of the effect of the posterior lens surface. As a consequence, phakic eyes become more hypermetropic when filled with silicone oil. Aphakic eyes become less hyperopic because of the convex anterior surface of the silicone oil. These changes after intravitreal silicone injection have a net effect of a shift toward myopia in aphakic eyes and toward hyperopia in phakic eyes after intravitreal silicone oil injection. A shift toward hyperopia occurred in 12 of 13 phakic eyes after intravitreal silicone injection,[15] with a mean shift of +5.57 diopters (D) in spherical equivalents (range, −2.38 to 10.38 D). After silicone injection in the six aphakic eyes, the mean shift was a spherical equivalent of −6.70 D (range, −2.63 to −9.50 D). In the 14 eyes that underwent lensectomy at the time of vitrectomy or later intracapsular cataract extraction, the mean shift was a spherical equivalent of −6.30 D (range, −1.25 to 18.38 D).[15]

The investigators[15] also found that positioning affected refraction. In 3 of 15 patients, a shift toward myopia, which was more pronounced in aphakic than in phakic patients, occurred when posturing changed from erect to supine. In a supine position, the silicone oil, which floats on aqueous, moves forward and separates from the retina. This produces a positive posterior oil surface that contributes toward the myopic shift. In phakic patients, the lens prevents any change in the curvature of the anterior surface of the silicone oil, whereas in aphakic patients, the oil can move forward through the pupil to increase the anterior convexity of the surface. This results in more of a myopic shift in aphakic than in phakic patients.

A reduced ability to accommodate was found in the five prepresbyopic phakic eyes in the study after intravitreal silicone oil injection. The investigators[15] speculated that this reduced ability might be caused by early cataract formation.

In 1958, Stone[16] reported that "various viscosities of silicone" injected into the vitreous cavity of rabbits produced no change in rabbit eyes over a 2-year period. He indicated that, because silicone is available in various viscosities, one with the precise viscosity should maintain the clarity of the vitreous and help reposition the retina while prohibiting seepage through a retinal tear. After Stone's initial work, a number of investigators began using silicone experimentally and clinically to treat retinal detachment. In a series of reports since 1962, Cibis and co-workers described using a silicone (viscosity, 1,000 cSt) injection combined with subretinal drainage both experimentally and clinically.[9,17-19] They used a special blunt-ended syringe to inject silicone into the preretinal space and achieved success in many cases of PVR that were previously considered hopeless or inoperable. Cibis and co-workers concluded that the use of silicone, although not without complications, offered hope in otherwise hopeless cases.[19] Similar experiences using silicones were reported by Armaly in 1962[20] and by a number of other investigators.[21-23]

Interest in the use of silicone to treat complicated retinal detachments diminished in the 1970s with the development of vitrectomy instrumentation and reports of silicone's adverse effects.[5,23-28] However, the surgical success rate using vitrectomy, membrane peeling, and intraocular gas to treat PVR was poor.[29] Other reports have refuted earlier evidence of silicone's toxicity[16,30-32] and have suggested that many complications associated with its use could be avoided with proper surgical technique.[33] Also described were favorable results in eyes considered to be inoperable by other methods.[33-35] These reports have initiated a new interest in the use of silicone.

Until recently, the use of silicone oil has been limited to complex retinal detachments, in which conventional vitreoretinal surgery has resulted in a poor surgical success rate. These conditions include nontraumatic retinal detachment with PVR, severe diabetic traction retinal detachment, giant retinal tears, and traumatic retinal detachments with PVR. Silicone oil is currently being used as a short-term tamponade in the repair of eyes with large, multiple, or posterior breaks, eyes with retinal detachments caused by macular holes, and eyes considered to be at high risk for developing PVR because of redetachment with open breaks after unsuccessful retinal detachment surgery without vitrectomy.[6]

COMPLICATIONS OF SILICONE OIL USE

The main intraoperative problem involving silicone injection occurs when silicone gains access to the subretinal space through a preexisting retinal tear or hole.[23] This complication may be avoided by closing retinal holes, by prior drainage of subretinal fluid, and by performing air–fluid exchange and laser coagulation initially. Should silicone gain access to the subretinal space, air should be replaced with fluid and the silicone aspirated through an anteriorly located hole.

Removal of traction around retinal tears before intravitreal injections also minimizes these complications. Occasionally, subretinal silicone may be removed by making a partial retinotomy and aspirating the bubble through the retinal breech, using a short plastic cannula. Silicone oil adheres to plastic but is repelled by metal. With the patient supine, subretinal silicone usually floats to a peripheral position and remains there because of the pressure of the intraocular silicone oil tamponade. Removal may involve the creation of a peripheral retinotomy, followed by suction with a plastic cannula.

Silicone oil is removed postoperatively to prevent the development or progression of intraocular complications or to reverse those complications.[11,12] In a series[36] involving silicone oil removal from 120 consecutive eyes after a mean of 30 weeks, postoperative retinal detachment occurred in 19% of eyes. Visual acuity improved in most eyes after silicone oil removal. Factors contributing to improvement in vision included removal of silicone oil emulsification, cataract extraction, and the absence of optical effects caused by the silicone oil bubble. Although nearly all eyes eventually developed cataracts, the rate of progression was slowed when silicone oil was removed before 12 weeks.[36]

Complications after silicone oil injection can be divided into early and late phases. Early complications are primarily limited to the anterior segment. Pang et al[37] studied 45 patients undergoing vitrectomy and intraocular silicone oil injection over a period of 13 months. Over a follow-up period averaging 8.5 months, they found irreversible silicone keratopathy in 50% of eyes undergoing pars plana lensectomy, vitrectomy, and intravitreal injection of silicone oil. In these eyes, no capsule or lens was present to prevent the anterior migration of silicone oil. In patients undergoing only a pars plana vitrectomy with intravitreal injection of silicone oil, 60% developed a cataract by 8 weeks. Thirty-three (40% of each group) developed a transient increase in intraocular pressure (IOP), which was well controlled with medications. Iritis also was present in these eyes.[37]

Late complications attributed to silicone oil injection include cataract, glaucoma, keratopathy, iritis, endophthalmitis, and recurrent retinal detachment.[23,38,39] Inflammatory surface silicone membranes have been found to occur as both early and late complications after intravitreal silicone oil injection.[33,39]

Retinal Tolerance and Toxicity

Since the introduction of silicone oil as an internal tamponading agent in the treatment of complicated retinal detachment, various histopathologic effects on ocular structures have been described after silicone oil injection in animal and human eyes.

In a series of related experiments using owl monkey eyes, Mukai and colleagues[28,40] and Lee et al[41] injected silicone oil in the posterior vitreous. These investigators reported the presence of vacuoles in the photoreceptor cells, ganglion cells, and corneal endothelium, along with nerve fiber layer swelling and ganglion layer degeneration. Other investigators demonstrated the presence of small silicone oil vacuoles in the retina, optic nerve, anterior chamber angle, corneal endothelium, and iris stroma.[25,42-51] Aggregates of macrophages engulfing silicone oil globules were reported by Shields and Eagle[52] on the surface of the retina, ciliary body, and trabecular meshwork in an eye enucleated 2 years after silicone oil injection. Ober and associates,[31] studying eyes 3 months after intravitreal silicone oil injection, reported only mild vacuolation of the inner limiting membrane, whereas Parmley and associates,[50] in a histologic study of an eye enucleated 20 months after vitrectomy and intraocular silicone injection, observed a foreign body giant cell reaction. Clear small vacuoles present in clusters were demonstrated in the anterior chamber angle and iris stroma. In contrast, other studies[20,32,53,54] have failed to demonstrate any morphologic retinal changes, contradicting the observation that silicone oil has a toxic effect on the retina.

Experiments by Ober and colleagues[31] support the lack of retinotoxicity of silicone. After vitrectomy, 14 rabbits received intravitreal injections of 0.75 to 1.5 mL liquid silicone (1,000 cSt); in 12 rabbits, the other eye was injected with balanced salt solution (BSS), and two eyes served as controls. Photopic and mesopic electroretinograms (ERGs) performed at 3-month and 6-month intervals after injection were normal in both groups of eyes. Armaly[20] also was unable to document ERG changes in eyes after silicone injection.

In contrast, Meredith et al, in 1985,[55] noted reduction of the a-wave and b-wave amplitude in the ERG of vitrectomized pigmented rabbit eyes that had received intravitreal silicone in the early postoperative period and had shown no deterioration, even 20 months later. This finding indicated that there was no accumulated toxic effect from silicone oil left in the eye for long periods. Thaler et al,[56] in 1986, noted, in their ERG and electrooculogram (EOG) recordings in patients immediately before, soon after, and up to 4 months after removal of silicone oil, that the amplitude (in ERG) and the standing potential (in EOG) increased after silicone oil removal. Similar results were reported by Foerster et al 1985.[57] Momirov and associates, in 1983,[58] noted lower recording potentials in eyes with silicone oil and also that the amount of decreased amplitude in the ERG is related to the amount of silicone oil injected.

Scott[33] concluded that ERG changes recorded in monkeys after intraocular silicone injection by both Lee and associates[41] and Mukai and co-workers[40] were caused by the insulating properties of silicone.

In a series of experiments, silicone oil was found to extract the lipophilic substances retinol and cholesterol from the retina.[59] In vitro experiments involving calf retinas exposed to silicone demonstrated by fluoroscopic spectroscopy retinol and cholesterol dissolved in the silicone. Further studies on cat and human eyes after vitrectomy demonstrated colorimetrically both retinol and cholesterol dissolved in silicone removed from these eyes, whereas analysis of fluid from control eyes gave negative results for the presence of these two lipophilic substances. Silicone oil removed from human eyes at 51 weeks and 96 weeks postoperatively contained cholesterol. This experiment suggests that silicone oils are not inert but can extract lipid substances from the retina. The investigators conclude that the effect on vision resulting from extraction of these two lipophilic substances is unknown, and the results of these tests do not mean that silicone oil is toxic.

Both gross and electron microscopic studies failed to demonstrate signs of retinal toxicity, except for minor changes probably attributable to surgical trauma or fixation artifact. Clinical observations by Haut and associates[30] and Leaver and co-workers[60] support the lack of demonstrable retinotoxicity by silicone. Should retinal complications be observed, removal of liquid silicone is possible.

The contradictory nature of these reports suggests that the safety of long-term intraocular silicone oil remains unresolved. The use of silicone is reserved by many investigators for eyes with complicated retinal detachments, whereas gas is considered as effective in these eyes when a prolonged internal tamponade is not required. Many surgeons advocate removal of silicone oil after several months to prevent keratopathy, cataract formation, and other silicone-related complications.[36]

Emulsification

Emulsification is considered to be a major complication associated with intravitreal silicone oil use. Normally, when silicone oil is in contact with fluid, interfacial tension keeps both liquids immiscible and the silicone bubble whole.

Emulsification[1,4,5] involves the formation of silicone oil bubbles (Figs. 1–2,

1–3). These may form on the surface of ocular tissues or at the interface between silicone oil and intraocular fluids.[61] The interfacial tension refers to the forces between two immiscible substances. Surface tension affects emulsification.[12,61]

Small vacuoles presumably composed of silicone oil droplets have been observed on the iris surface, preretinal membranes, and throughout the retina, optic disc, and vitreous body.[62] In one study[38] of 150 eyes treated with silicone oil for complicated retinal detachments, these tiny silicone droplets were observed on the anterior lens capsule, on the posterior iris surface, in the superior angle, on and between the ciliary process, on the zonules, on the epiretinal surface, and on the retroretinal surface in some cases with detached retina.

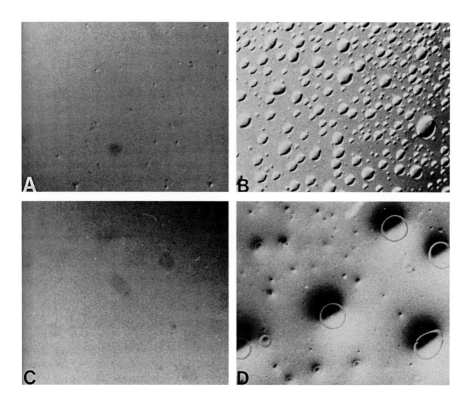

Figure 1–2. Phase-contrast photomicrographs ($\times$ 100) demonstrating effect of benzalkonium chloride with varying concentrations of fetal bovine serum (FBS) on emulsification of silicone oil (1,000 cSt, Dow Corning 360). **A.** No FBS, no emulsification observed. **B.** 10% FBS, prominent stable emulsification. Oil bubbles are relatively uniform and dispersed in aqueous phase. **C.** 40% FBS, no emulsification. Oil bubbles are relatively uniform and dispersed in aqueous phase. **D.** 100% FBS, moderate dispersion of oil bubbles in aqueous phase. Bubbles vary greatly in size and are unstable (i.e., will rapidly separate in bulk phases). (From Crisp A, de Juan E Jr, Tiedeman J: Effect of silicone oil viscosity on emulsification. *Arch Ophthalmol* 1987;105:546–550. Copyright, American Medical Association.)

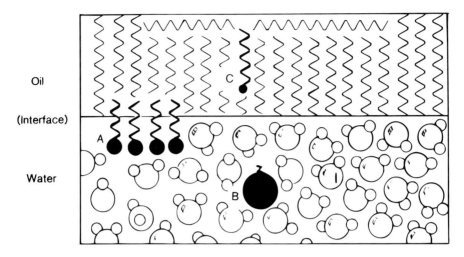

Figure 1–3. Effect of molecular composition on ability of molecule to function as surface-active agent (emulsifier). Darker jagged lines represent oil-soluble (nonpolar) portion of emulsifier, and dark circles represent polar or hydrophilic part of compound. Both polar and nonpolar regions must be present for molecule to function as emulsifier (**A**). If compound is too polar or too nonpolar (**B** and **C**, respectively), it will not function as an effective emulsifier. (From Crisp A, de Juan E Jr, Tiedeman J: Effect of silicone oil viscosity on emulsification. *Arch Ophthalmol* 1987,105.546–550. Copyright, American Medical Assocation.)

Emulsification facilitates migration of silicone oil into the anterior chamber, where mechanical contact with the cornea may result in keratopathy and obstructions of the trabecular meshwork, causing glaucoma.[30,61] Silicone droplets may gain access to the subretinal space through retinal tears, thus interfering with retinal re-attachment.[12,61] Silicone droplets in the vitreous cavity may interfere with examination of the retina.[25,61] When located in the optic axis, they may interfere with the patient's vision.[25,61]

In one large series of eyes with intravitreal silicone oil, some degree of emulsification was demonstrated by 1% of eyes at the 1-month follow-up, by 6% at 2 months, 11% at 3 months, 85% at 6 months, and 100% at 12 months. Five months was the mean time for development of emulsification in these eyes.[38]

The interfacial tension that keeps silicone immiscible can be overcome by surface active agents or by emulsifiers, including various components of plasma, proteinaceous agents, different impurities, and phospholipids from red blood cells. Surface tension causes silicone oil in contact with a liquid to form the smallest surface area–volume ratio. Eye movement may impart mechanical energy, which interferes with interfacial energy and increases the surface area, leading to emulsification.[1,2,4,5]

Chemical composition and stability determine the susceptibility of silicone oil to emulsification. Besides physicochemical properties, the stability of silicone oil also is affected by the presence of biologic detergents.

Interfacial tensions were found to contribute to emulsification, with lower tensions predisposing to more emulsification. Interfacial tension increases as the viscosity of silicone oil increases. When comparing silicone oil and fluorosilicone oil of the same viscosity, silicone oil was less emulsified. The investigators postulated that silicone oil and intraocular fluids are closer in density than fluorosilicone oils and water, which makes agitation of silicone oil more difficult.[1]

Crisp and associates[1] demonstrated that silicone oil with higher viscosity composed of homogeneous long chains resisted emulsification better than did low-viscosity oils composed of homogeneous LMWCs. Removal of LMWCs allows the silicone oil to better resist emulsification (Fig. 1–4).

Previous studies by Heidenkummer and associates[63,64] found little difference in stability between silicone oils with viscosities of 5,000 cSt and 10,000 cSt. Little difference existed in the tendency to emulsify among silicone oils with viscosities ranging from 5,000 to 10,000 cSt, although a notable difference existed among silicone oils with viscosities varying from 1,000 to 5,000 cSt. In a more recent study[65] comparing silicone oils with viscosities between 1,000 cSt and 5,000 cSt, no positive correlation was found between emulsification and increases in viscosity from the 1,000-cSt silicone to the intermediate group with viscosities between 2,000 cSt and 4,000 cSt. The markedly diminished extent and susceptibility of the 5,000-cSt silicone oil to emulsification was explained on the basis of molecular entanglement, with the investigators suggesting that highly purified silicone oils with a viscosity below 5,000 cSt be used in vitreoretinal surgery. The tendency of highly viscous long chains of silicone polymers to become physically entangled in loops of other chains is postulated to limit both the movement of one molecule relative to neighboring molecules and the penetration of solute detergents into highly viscous silicones.[1]

In the absence of reduced surface tension, eye movement is not usually considered to have the ability to cause small silicone oil droplets to break away from the oil bubble inside the eye. Besides requiring shearing forces created by rotational and shaking actions, the presence of substances in the aqueous phase lowers the surface tension usually necessary for purified silicone oil to emulsify. The small bubbles of silicone that may result from ocular movement in the absence of surface tension–lowering agents coalesce eventually into the main silicone oil bubble.[64,66]

Heidenkummer et al[64] demonstrated that fibrin and serum are strong biologically active emulsifiers. Additional biologic emulsifiers include gamma-globulins, acidic alpha-1-glycoproteins, and very-low-density lipoproteins (VLDL). The investigators noted that, in the presence of ionic solutions, the biologic emulsifiers are able to accelerate and destabilize intraocular silicone oils.

Bartov et al[66] experimentally evaluated several substances for emulsification potential. Marked emulsification was induced by ghost red blood cells, but hemoglobin and red blood cells had a low emulsifying effect. However, the hemoglobin tested was a hypotonic solution. Consequently, it may have a greater emulsifying effect under normotonic conditions. Various other plasma components, including lymphocytes and plasma, also induced significant emulsification.

Platelets, in contrast to other plasma components, had minimal effect on silicone oil emulsification. The investigators[66] concluded that, because various compo-

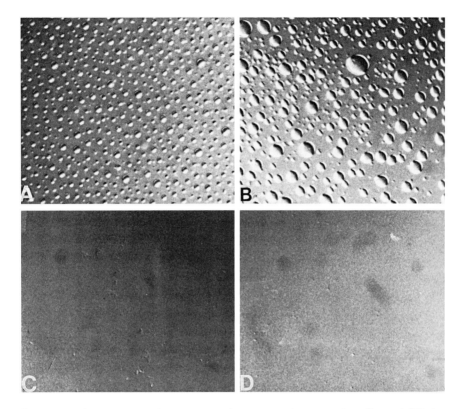

Figure 1–4. Phase-contrast photomicrographs ($\times$ 100) demonstrating effects of differing viscosity and molecular composition silicone oils in an in vitro model of silicone oil emulsification. **A.** 100 cSt, highly stable and uniform emulsion of oil in aqueous phase. **B.** 1,000 cSt (Medical 380, Dow Corning), stable but less uniform emulsion of oil. **C.** 1,000 cSt (Wacker), no emulsification. **D.** 12,500 cSt (Dow Corning), no emulsification. (From Crisp A, de Juan E Jr, Tiedeman J: Effect of silicone oil viscosity on emulsification. *Arch Ophthalmol* 1987;105:546–550. Copyright, American Medical Association.)

nents of blood carried significant silicone emulsification, any intravitreal blood accumulating during surgery should be meticulously removed, and attempts should be made to minimize hemorrhage surgically in eyes that contain silicone oil as a tamponading agent. Frequent postoperative observation of eyes containing silicone was recommended, with prompt, aggressive treatment of any intraocular inflammation.

Perisilicone Membrane

Lewis and associates[67] reported a series of 31 eyes undergoing silicone oil injection, of which 19 developed cell proliferation, ultimately causing recurrent retinal detachment in 15 eyes (49%). These membranes were apparent at an average of 5 weeks after surgery.

Reproliferation on the retinal surface after intravitreal silicone oil injection occurred in 23 (15.3%) of the 150 silicone-filled eyes reported by Federman and Schubert.[38] Reproliferation caused by compartmentalization was originally described by Charles.[68] The postoperative reproliferation frequently associated with recurrent tractional retinal detachment occurs in areas in which the tamponading agent is not in contact with the retina. As a lighter-than-water vitreous substitute, silicone provides a superior retinal tamponade, but because a total vitreous cavity fill is impossible, a residual fluid space exists in the inferior retina. Mitogens and chemoattractants, as well as inflammatory mediators and serum components that stimulate PVR, are concentrated in the small aqueous spaces between the vitreous and retina, causing and accelerating reproliferation-enhancing membrane formation.[67,69,70]

Epiretinal reproliferation occurred either inferiorly or from the edges of retinotomies. Subretinal fibrous tissue formation occurred only in eyes with persistent subretinal fluid and in the areas where the fluid was located.[38]

Cataract

In the literature, the rate of cataract formation when silicone oil is used has varied between 78% and 100%. Most investigators believe the basis for cataract formation in silicone oil–filled eyes is mechanical rather than toxic. The diffusion of nutrients and other substances necessary for lens function is prevented by the silicone oil bubble.[71]

Federman and Schubert[38] reported that cataracts developed in all 33 phakic eyes in their series of 150 patients after successful reattachment of the retina with a silicone oil tamponade. Other investigators[27,39,72] noted that the rapidity of cataract formation is proportional to the duration of silicone oil contact with the lens. In contrast, Franks and Leaver[36] noted removal of silicone oil by 12 weeks delayed but did not prevent cataract formation.

In another study, Casswell and Gregor[73] found that lens opacities progressed in 85% of patients. Clinically significant cataracts developed in 60% of lenses that were clear at the time of silicone oil removal. In 13 eyes with established uncontrollable glaucoma, removal of silicone oil was combined with filtering surgery, resulting in control of IOP in all 13. In the nine patients with corneal involvement, eight improved or were unchanged after silicone oil removal. Three of these eyes also underwent successful keratoplasty with maintenance of clear grafts. Additionally, removal of silicone oil prevented the development of keratopathy or glaucoma in patients with these complications at the time of silicone removal.

Keratopathy

Sternberg and associates[74] noted that similar corneal morphologic changes were observed after injection of silicone, air, or gas into the anterior chamber of cats and rabbits (Figs. 1–5, 1–6). Based on these findings, the investigators postulated that many of the corneal changes were caused by a mechanical barrier effect rather than by a direct toxic effect of silicone oil on the corneal endothelium.

The stromal thinning in rabbits reported by Sternberg et al[74] and later observed clinically by Beekhuis et al[75] has been attributed to evaporation of water from the corneal surface, resulting in dehydration. Silicone oil provides a barrier that prevents aqueous from entering the corneal stroma. On removal of the silicone, corneal decompensation permitted rapid stromal and epithelial swelling. This finding was attributed to damaged and malfunctioning endothelial cells that permitted access to the stroma.

The development of silicone oil keratopathy (Fig. 1–7) primarily occurs in aphakic eyes, usually after prolonged and extensive contact between a silicone oil bubble and the corneal endothelium.[76] Yet Setälä et al[77] demonstrated that even transient corneal endothelial contact with small droplets of silicone oil may contribute to the development of keratopathy. Corneal changes frequently present as bullous keratopathy in older patients, whereas younger patients are more likely to develop band keratopathy.[76] Biomicroscopy[78] and pachymetry determination may be used in eyes with severe corneal damage. Pachymetry is a more reliable method to detect early corneal change.[79]

Gao and associates[79] described 72 eyes with visible amounts of silicone oil in the anterior chamber after pars plana vitrectomy. Despite the removal of silicone oil from the anterior chamber in 30 eyes, nearly two thirds of the eyes in the series developed silicone oil keratopathy. This high rate of corneal decompensation emphasizes the importance of frequent ocular examinations and prompt removal of any silicone oil discovered in the anterior chamber.

Additional reports[73,75,77-80] suggested that aqueous flow into the stroma is obstructed by silicone oil adherent to the corneal endothelium. This mechanical effect results in corneal endothelial dysfunction from hypoxia and lack of nutrition.[80]

Other investigators[76,81] supported this concept by noting that the degree of corneal clarity in silicone oil–filled eyes is frequently not representative of the corneal endothelial damage present.

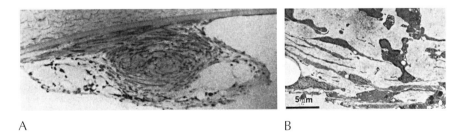

A   B

Figure 1–5. A. Light photomicrograph of retrocorneal membrane at edge of silicone oil bubble after 3 weeks in cat (azure II and methylene blue, × 350). **B.** Transmission electron micrograph of posterior surface of same retrocorneal membrane. Clear spaces probably contained silicone oil (× 3,500). (From Sternberg P Jr, Hatchell DL, Foulks GN, et al: The effect of silicone oil on the cornea. *Arch Ophthalmol* 1985;103:90–94.)

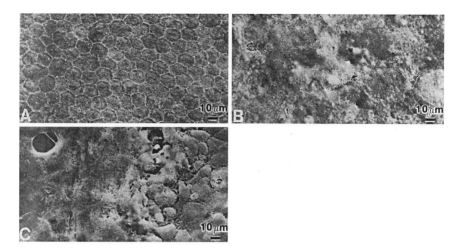

Figure 1–6. Scanning electron micrographs of rabbit cornea. **A.** Normal endothelial cells outside area of silicone–endothelial contact (× 400). **B.** Connective tissue layer on posterior surface of cornea that had been in contact with oil (× 400). **C.** Retrocorneal membrane in transition zone at edge of bubble (× 400). (From Sternberg P Jr, Hatchell DL, Foulks GN, et al: The effect of silicone oil on the cornea. *Arch Ophthalmol* 1985;103:90–94.)

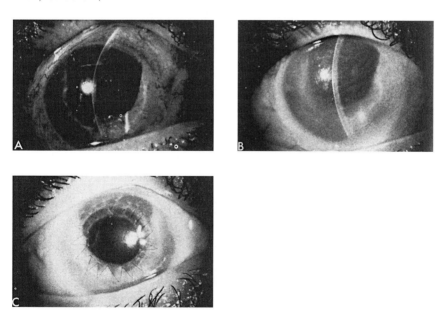

Figure 1–7. Silicone keratopathy. **A.** Anterior segment 3 weeks after silicone oil injection for PVR. Silicone fills the anterior chamber. **B.** Silicone keratopathy 4 months after silicone oil injection. **C.** Appearance of anterior segment 6 months after removal of silicone oil and penetrating keratoplasty. (From McCuen BW II, De Juan E Jr, Landers MB III, et al: Silicone oil in vitreoretinal surgery: Part 2. Results and complications. *Retina* 1985;5:198–205.)

Surgical methods that minimize prolapse of silicone into the anterior chamber include avoiding overfill of the eye with silicone oil, using the correct amount of silicone oil, maintaining a normal IOP at the completion of the surgery, and filling the anterior chamber with air in aphakic eyes before silicone oil injection.[79]

Silicone-induced corneal damage may be reduced by creating an inferior iridectomy in aphakic eyes (Fig. 1–8), which prevents pupillary block formation frequently caused by prolapse of silicone into the anterior chamber. Additionally, prompt repair of retinal detachment is required because this condition is associated with the late appearance of silicone oil in the anterior chamber caused by shrinkage of intravitreal volume.

In a separate series[38] involving complications after silicone oil injection, with a mean follow-up period of 31.6 months, peripheral iridectomies performed in 90 of the 105 eyes remained patent and functional. Silicone oil was immediately removed in the other 15 eyes with closure of the inferior iridectomy. Despite forward displacement of silicone oil, all keratopathy was avoided by prompt silicone oil removal.

Madreperla and McCuen[82] evaluated the effect of closure of a surgical inferior peripheral iridectomy on silicone oil position in aphakic eyes treated with a silicone oil extended tamponade. Eighty-seven eyes were included in this retrospective study, with a follow-up period of 12 months if possible. The rate of closure was highest for eyes with proliferative diabetic retinopathy (60%). In contrast, 28% of eyes with PVR experienced iridectomy closure during follow-up. Iris neovascularization and the tendency toward fibrin membrane formation are factors associated with the high incidence of iridectomy closure in patients with proliferative diabetic retinopathy.

The rate of corneal touch for eyes with open peripheral iridectomies was 9.8% versus 80% of those with closed peripheral iridectomies.[82] The investigators concluded that, given the irreversible nature of the keratopathy associated with corneal touch, maintaining a patent iridectomy is extremely important.

Complications associated with silicone oil in the anterior chamber are diminished by opening the peripheral iridectomy with laser or other techniques.[82]

In diabetic patients with fibrin membranes unresponsive to antiinflammatory treatment because of closure of the iridectomy, the use of lasers or other treatment (tissue plasminogen activator) is justified.[82]

In a separate report, Zumbro and associates[83] used an in vitro model to demonstrate that the presence of silicone oil in the posterior chamber diminished the effectiveness of the neodymium: yttrium aluminum garnet (Nd:YAG) laser in creating an iridotomy. Fewer holes were created when the viscosity of the silicone oil increased while the thickness of the membrane and Nd:YAG energy levels remained constant.[83]

The presence of a large superior iridectomy or sector iridectomy also may allow silicone oil to enter the anterior chamber. Subsequently, prophylactic closure of a large superior iridectomy with iris suturing before filling the eye with silicone may be indicated to prevent forward movement of silicone into the anterior chamber.[76]

The use of the Nd:YAG laser has been described in the silicone oil–filled eye.[84]

Huy et al[85] noted that exposure in vitro of silicone to radiation from Nd:YAG

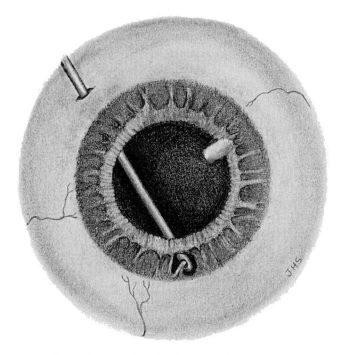

Figure 1–8. Alternative method (Ando) of making an inferior iridectomy for PVR silicone implantation.

photodisruption results in the formation of gas bubbles. Breakage of the Si–C bonds in the silicone oil probably results in the formation of silica and transient volatile hydrocarbon gases, primarily ethylene, methane, and traces of ethane. The silica microfibrillae, by depositing on the retina, theoretically could affect vision, and breakage of the Si–O bonds could modify the silicone oil viscosity. Both events are extremely unlikely to be of clinical significance. Local transient oxygen depletion could result from production of the three hydrocarbon gases, but again, any damage from the process is doubtful.

Glaucoma

After cataract, postoperative glaucoma is the second most common complication in patients who have been injected with intravitreal silicone oil (Fig. 1–9).[35,42,86,87] In 1967, Watzke[25] reported the occurrence of postoperative glaucoma after intravitreal silicone oil injection but pointed out that the presence of intraocular silicone in the anterior chamber was not the only cause of increased IOP. In 1977, Grey and Leaver[35] found silicone bubbles in the anterior chamber angle of patients with increased IOP but noticed no difference in the incidence of glaucoma in phakic and aphakic patients. Leaver and co-workers[86] reported that 43% of the patients with postoperative glaucoma had silicone oil bubbles in the anterior chamber angle. Haut and co-workers[30] described similar findings in their previous series. Alexandridis and Daniel[87] observed that the incidence of postoperative glaucoma was more common in aphakic eyes. Laroche and co-workers[46] reported glaucoma as a late complication of silicone oil injection but questioned whether it was caused by the presence of silicone oil in the angle.

In the past, an early postoperative complication in aphakic eyes filled with silicone was ocular hypertension. Ando[88] recommended the creation of an inferior peripheral iridectomy to avoid this complication. The iridectomy, performed at the end of surgery before silicone oil injection, must be wide enough to avoid becoming plugged by inflammatory cells.

The inferior iridectomy allows aqueous access to the anterior chamber. In eyes with only a superior iridectomy, the silicone oil floats on aqueous and is easily able to block this opening and herniate into the anterior chamber. When the patient is supine, aqueous flows behind the silicone oil bubble and pushes the bubble forward until pupillary block develops. The anterior chamber either becomes totally filled with silicone or the iris is pressed against the cornea to close the angle completely. Intraocular pressure increases in both instances.[89]

Postoperatively, the inferior iridectomy may become occluded because of fibrin deposits and result in an elevated IOP. If treatment of the intraocular inflammation fails, steroids may reopen the iridectomy; and if the IOP is excessively high, the iridectomy may need to be reopened with laser or surgery.[90]

In aphakic patients, an inferior iridectomy also may close because of capsular remnants that remain in the eye. Reopening of the iridectomy using the YAG laser or a surgical iridectomy is necessary. Federman and Schubert[38] noted that, in 15 (14.5%) of the 105 aphakic eyes filled with silicone, the iridectomy was closed as a result of inflammation, pigment cell proliferation in the inferior angle, or rubeosis. Complete removal of the lens capsule may prevent reproliferation and subsequent closure of the iridectomy.

A mechanical overfill of silicone oil also can lead to pupillary block glaucoma. The only treatment is removal of the excess silicone.

Silicone-induced pupillary block has been described in a phakic eye where a small zonulysis allowed silicone to enter the anterior chamber during surgery. After surgery, a pupillary block was created by the anterior flow of silicone. The involved eye had an excessively deep posterior chamber filled with silicone, whereas the iris was nearly pressed against the cornea. The investigators recommend performing an inferior iridectomy in phakic eyes when silicone oil is found in the anterior chamber at the time of surgery.[91]

Choroidal detachment may cause forward displacement of silicone oil in aphakic eyes, resulting in pupillary block glaucoma. Management consists of draining choroidal detachment and replacing the silicone oil with a long-acting gas.[38]

Emulsification of silicone oil with droplets entering the trabecular meshwork may interfere with the intraocular fluid flow. A glaucoma refractive to medical treatment may result from these silicone oil deposits.[64]

Moisseiev et al[92] noted that removal of emulsified silicone more than 6 months after injection failed to control IOP in 10 of 11 eyes with glaucoma. Severe deterio-

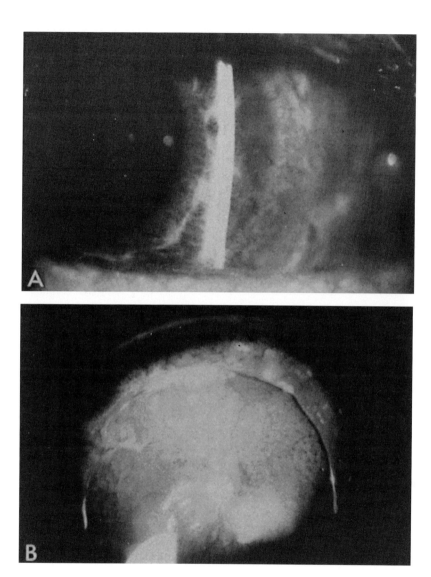

Figure 1–9. Glaucoma after silicone oil injection. **A.** Acute angle closure glaucoma 1 day after silicone oil injection caused by silicone-induced pupillary block. **B.** "Emulsification" of silicone oil with tiny silicone bubbles present superiorly just posterior to the encircling buckle. (From McCuen BW II, De Juan E Jr, Landers MB III, et al: Silicone oil in vitreoretinal surgery: Part 2. Results and complications. *Retina* 1985;5:198–205.)

ration of visual acuity in these eyes with glaucoma occurred during the 12-month period after silicone oil removal. These results suggest that late removal of emulsified silicone oil fails to control glaucoma.[92]

Because vitrectomy also can produce glaucoma by different mechanisms[93] in many eyes, especially after multiple procedures, the development of glaucoma cannot always be attributed to the intravitreal injection of silicone. Instead, the causes may be multifactorial, including rubeosis iridis, erythroclastic causes, hemolytic causes, mechanical conditions (hemorrhage or silicone oil bubbles), inflammation, phagolytic causes, response to steroids, and pupillary block.[93] We conclude that all of these factors may contribute to the elevation of IOP in patients who have been injected with intravitreal silicone oil.[94]

Nguyen and associates[95] reported medically uncontrollable glaucoma occurred postoperatively in 21 (42%) of 50 eyes after intravitreal silicone oil injection for complicated retinal detachment. Fourteen eyes underwent silicone oil removal, and normal IOP was reestablished in eight eyes. Glaucoma surgery was performed on seven eyes, including three after silicone oil removal. Filtering procedures, which carry an extremely poor prognosis in eyes with previous multiple procedures, were avoided in favor of glaucoma shunt implants or cyclodestructive procedures. Control of IOP was achieved in one eye after Nd:YAG transscleral cyclophotocoagulation and in three of five eyes undergoing Molteno shunt implantation. The IOP remained elevated in one eye after a modified Schocket procedure.

Compared with earlier reports on the use of silicone oil in eyes with PVR in which a 15% prevalence of elevated IOP was noted, recent studies have documented a lower incidence of glaucoma. The Silicone Study[96] noted a chronically elevated IOP in 11 of 241 eyes (5%) with severe PVR (C_3 or worse). Eyes randomized to silicone oil had a higher incidence of chronic glaucoma compared with eyes in the C_3F_8 gas group (8% versus 2%). The investigators suggest that the decrease in prevalence of glaucoma in silicone oil–filled eyes is attributable to several factors, including the use of pure silicone of low molecular weight from which contaminants have been removed, minimizing droplet formation; the creation of an inferior iridectomy in all aphakic eyes, which diminishes the displacement of silicone into the anterior chamber and reduces the incidence of pupillary block glaucoma; and the removal of silicone from eyes with normal IOP, which may prevent a later pressure increase.

Retinal Detachment After Oil Removal

In 85 eyes undergoing vitrectomy and silicone oil exchange for PVR or giant retinal tears, the major complications of silicone oil removal were retinal detachment (25%, Fig. 1–10), hypotony (16%), and expulsive hemorrhage (1%).[73]

In a multicenter, randomized clinical trial[97] that compared the effectiveness of silicone oil and sulfur hexafluoride gas (SF_6) as tamponading agents in 101 eyes with rhegmatogenous retinal detachment and severe PVR (grade C_3 or worse), recurrent retinal detachments developed in 14% (3) of 21 eyes immediately after removal of silicone oil. A related study involving 265 eyes with rhegmatogenous retinal detachment and severe PVR (grade C_3 or worse) treated with silicone oil or perfluoro-

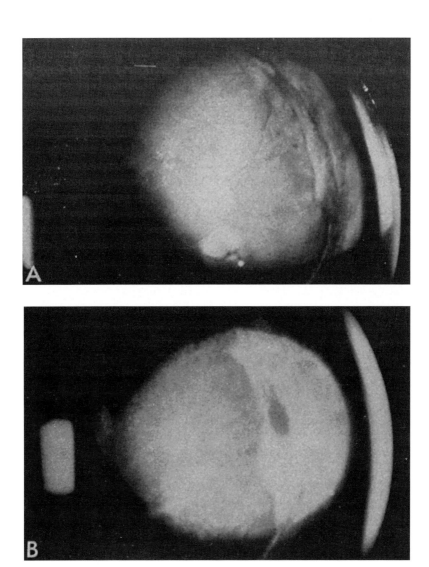

Figure 1–10. Recurrent retinal detachment with reproliferation after silicone oil injection. **A.** Fundus appearance 6 weeks after silicone oil injection for PVR. **B.** Fundus of same eye 4 months after silicone oil injection with the development of reproliferation and tractional retinal detachment nasally. (From McCuen BW II, De Juan E Jr, Landers MB III, et al: Silicone oil in vitreoretinal surgery: Part 2. Results and complications. *Retina* 1985;5:198–205.)

propane gas (C_3F_8) as tamponading agents had similar results. Immediately after removal of silicone oil, recurrent retinal detachment developed in 8% (3) of 36 eyes that had previously undergone vitrectomy and in 3% (1) of 33 eyes that had not previously been vitrectomized. At last follow-up examination, macular detachment after silicone oil removal was found in 8% (4) of the group of vitrectomized eyes and in 9% (3) of the group of eyes that had not undergone previous vitrectomy.

These and similar results[76,98-100] suggest that silicone oil removal might be associated with retinal detachment.

Proliferative vitreoretinopathy is the most common cause of failure of retinal detachment surgery. Reproliferation of membranes is usually the cause of retinal detachment in eyes in which silicone oil has not been removed.[6,98] After silicone oil usage, the reported rate of retinal redetachment has varied from 9% to 30%.[98,101,102] Lucke and Laqua[71] found in a large series of eyes that reproliferation was the main cause of redetachment after silicone oil removal in eyes that had undergone surgery for PVR.

Ando et al[103] suggested that the preretinal fibrous tissue should be removed in eyes with traction retinal detachment immediately after silicone oil removal.

Reproliferation in the posterior pole frequently is also a cause of retinal detachment after removal of silicone oil in diabetic eyes.[5,71]

Živojnović[5] reported that secondary hemorrhage, residual tissue, remnants of fibrovascular tissue, sites of previous vitreoretinal adhesions, and at times the edges of retinectomies and iatrogenic holes are the main sources of reproliferation. To prevent or minimize reproliferation before silicone oil injection, Živojnović advises accurate cautery of bleeding sites and careful removal of fibrovascular membranes.

Kampik and associates[104] noted that the risks associated with silicone oil removal were higher in eyes with proliferative diabetic retinopathy compared with those with PVR. The investigators suggest that the better outcome in proliferative diabetic retinopathy may be attributable to the absence of a PVR component in many eyes and the use of panretinal photocoagulation, which stabilizes the retina. Sixteen of 39 eyes with PVR developed retinal detachment after silicone oil removal, compared with 8 out of 36 eyes in the severe proliferative diabetic retinopathy group.

The second Silicone Study[105,106] emphasized the need for additional retinal reattachment surgery after removal of silicone oil in eyes in which vitrectomy was performed for advanced PVR. In 24 of 63 eyes with previous vitrectomy, the retina remained completely attached after silicone oil removal. Additionally, 13 of 19 eyes in this group required a total of 24 reoperations for a total anatomic success rate of 61%.

Subconjunctival Silicone Oil

In a series[38] reporting the complications of silicone oil after use in 150 eyes with complicated vitreoretinal problems, 2.7% (4 eyes) developed subconjunctival silicone oil. All four eyes with extravasation of silicone oil through the sclerotomy into the subconjunctival space presented with pain.

Hutchinson and associates[107] described an additional two patients with this complication. Both patients presented with a diffuse clear mass involving the bulbar conjunctiva, which coalesced after several weeks into firm transparent subepithelial droplets. Histopathologic examination of involved conjunctiva excised from one eye showed both intracellular and extracellular silicone oil droplets in the presence of fibrovascular tissue infiltrated with chronic inflammatory cells.

Hypotony

Results of the Silicone Study suggest that hypotony is a more important clinical problem than chronically elevated IOP. Chronic hypotony was present in 24% of eyes in the Silicone Study compared with 5% of eyes having chronically elevated IOP. Hypotony was apparently twice as prevalent in eyes randomized to C_3F_8 gas as those randomized to silicone oil (31% versus 18%). No difference existed between groups I (with no vitrectomy) and II (with prior vitrectomy) in the prevalence rates of chronic hypotony, with the exception of eyes randomized to perfluorocarbon gas versus silicone oil. Anatomic failure was associated with an increased prevalence of chronic hypotony (48% versus 16%). Univariate analysis demonstrated that preoperative retinal breaks greater than or equal to 2 disc diameters, preoperative rubeosis, and preoperative hypotony were factors predictive of postoperative chronic hypotony. Multivariate analysis demonstrated that a fourfold increase in the risk of chronic hypotony was present in eyes with diffuse contractions of retina anterior to the equator caused by the presence of an epiretinal membrane extending from the equator to the insertion of the posterior hyaloid. Stratified analysis indicated diffuse anterior contraction resulted in a 4 to 5 times greater risk of chronic hypotony regardless of the status of the retina.[96]

Additionally, the Silicone Study[96] demonstrated that the only operative factor associated with postoperative chronic hypotony was the use of perfluorocarbon gas. Operative parameters not associated with chronic hypotony included difficulty of membrane dissection, intraoperative complications, management of lens and iris, revision of the scleral buckle, and surgery duration. Postoperative correlates of postoperative chronic hypotony were retinal detachment, abnormal anterior chamber depth, poor visual acuity, and corneal opacities.

Theories as to the cause of hypotony in eyes with PVR include small dialysis clefts resulting from traction on the ciliary body, formation of a thin membrane in recurrent PVR that causes mechanical blockage of the ciliary processes, trauma damage to the ciliary processes, and repeated surgery resulting in mechanical damage to the ciliary processes.[96] The insulating effects of silicone oil have been postulated to result in hypotony caused by overcoagulation with cryotherapy.[96,108] No differences existed in the Silicone Study[96] in the adhesive modality (laser versus cryotherapy) used in eyes that developed chronic hypotony.

Inflammation

Johnson et al[109] demonstrated transient hypopyon with anterior chamber fibrin after pars plana vitrectomy and intravitreal silicone oil injection. Two of 30 patients undergoing surgery for complex retinal detachments developed marked postoperative anterior chamber fibrin and hypopyon. These two patients were treated with frequent topical steroids and antibiotics, and in both cases, clinical improvement and long-term retinal reattachment were achieved. The excessive postoperative inflammation was attributed to the intense scatter laser endophotocoagulation.[109] Federman and Schubert[38] reported a 0.7% incidence (one eye) of endophthalmitis in 150 eyes managed using pars plana vitrectomy with intravitreal silicone oil injection.[38]

INTRAOCULAR INJECTION OF SILICONE

In recent years, silicone oil has been injected intraocularly to treat complicated retinal detachment and PVR.[110-120] The silicone oil provides a prolonged tamponade of the retina, so that retinochoroidal adhesions have time to develop and counteract preretinal tractional forces. The silicone oil is often left inside the eye unless complications occur.[110,113]

The specific gravity of silicone is less than that of water and therefore provides a low buoyancy, which means that silicone does not press against the retinal surface nearly as thoroughly as an air or gas bubble.[12,121]

Silicone is preferable to air when used intraocularly because earlier visual rehabilitation of patients is possible. Additionally, the volume of silicone oil remains constant after intravitreal injection, which theoretically allows an indefinite retinal tamponade.[121]

Silicone oil can be injected intraocularly either by a gas–silicone exchange or by a direct fluid–silicone exchange. The advantages to the former procedures include better IOP control during the exchange, the reduced danger of silicone entering the subretinal space through a retinal hole, and the ability to use an established technique with only minor variations. The advantages of a direct silicone–fluid exchange are improved visualization, especially in phakic and pseudophakic eyes, and easily detected residual traction, because the retina slowly flattens.[121]

The two-stage procedure for silicone injection involves a modification of techniques used for a gas–fluid exchange (Fig. 1–11). A complete vitrectomy using a standard three-port system is carried out until all traction has been relieved. Any epiretinal membranes present are segmented and removed, if possible. After the vitreous suction cutter is removed, the infusion cannula is connected to an air pump system,[117,118] and a flute needle is introduced through the open sclerotomy to perform a complete air–fluid exchange. If any subretinal fluid is present, it can be drained internally at this time. Intraocular pressure is kept at approximately 40 mm Hg to maintain adequate expansion of the globe. After reattachment of the retina, any necessary endophotocoagulation is performed. The light pipe is removed, and the

Figure 1–11. A. Air–silicone exchange. Silicone oil enters into eye through an 18-gauge cannula, while air exits through the air infusion cannula. B. Air–silicone exchange continues until oil refluxes into the air infusion cannula. At this point, the cannula is clamped. The silicone oil bubble is behind the iris at the level of the sclerotomies.

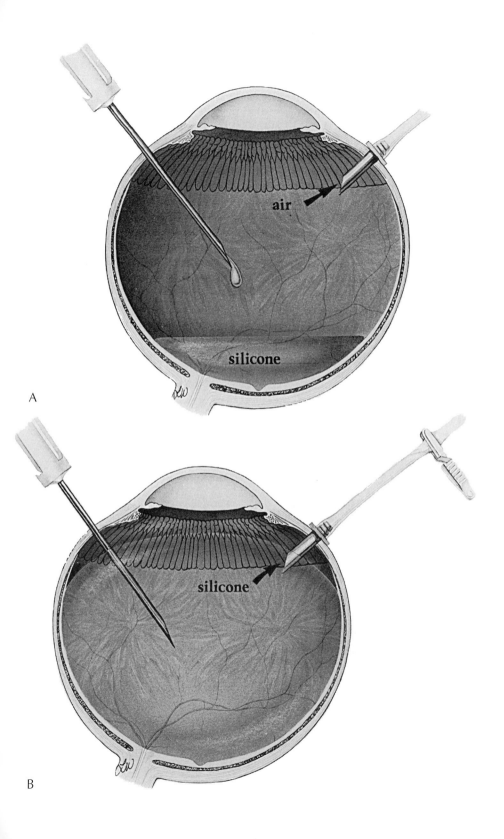

A

B

sclerotomy is closed securely with appropriate suture material. The flute needle is removed, and the sclerotomy is temporarily closed. When required, a scleral buckle is placed to relieve traction and to support the retina.

The force required to inject silicone oil intravitreally varies proportionately with viscosity. Viscous fluid injectors controlled by the surgeon with a foot pedal and the use of disposable syringes have been recommended for intravitreal silicone injection. These pumps either rely on an outside air pressure source or have a self-contained pump that holds the silicone being injected. Because pressures are greatest near the silicone container, and to prevent the tubing from becoming disconnected from the syringe, the injectors should have a locking syringe assembly.[121,122] Alternatively, silicone oil with a viscosity of 1,000 to 2,000 cSt has been injected intravitreally with a syringe attached directly to the infusion line of a short 20-gauge cannula[123] or a regular 18- or 20-gauge needle[108] placed through a sclerotomy port. High-viscosity silicone, such as the 12,500-cSt silicone tested by Grisolano and Peyman,[124] is more difficult to inject. Much resistance to flow occurs when the oil is injected through long- or small-bore needles. To facilitate injection, they advocated the use of short needles made by cutting standard, disposable 18-gauge needles to 6 mm and then placing a 45°, 2-mm bevel on the tip (Fig. 1–12). These short needles avoid retinal damage because they can be placed into the eye after the 20-gauge sclerotomy is widened with an MVR (microvitreoretinal) blade.

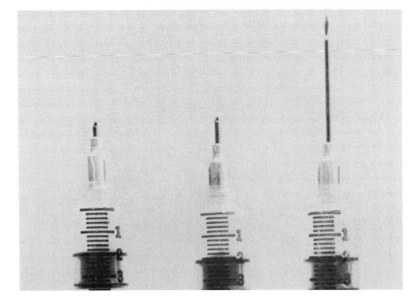

Figure 1–12. Standard 10-mL syringes are used with 16-gauge needles of different lengths. From left to right, 4-mm, 8-mm, and 4-cm needles. Only the short needles are recommended for silicone injection. (From Grisolano J, Peyman GA: Special short needles to inject and aspirate high-viscosity silicone oil. *Arch Ophthalmol* 1986;104:608.)

When compared with a syringe, the viscous fluid injectors give the surgeon more control over the amount of silicone injected intravitreally and prevent undesirable variations in IOP during injections, which can cause complications.

For manual injection of silicone, a short (5 to 6 mm long), blunt-tipped needle with an internal diameter of 16 or 18 gauge is used.[125] This needle is connected to a 10-mL syringe containing approximately 6 mL silicone oil and is introduced through the temporarily closed sclerotomy. Intraocular pressure is gradually lowered to approximately 10 mm Hg, using an air pump.[121,125]

A silicone–air exchange is performed with silicone entering the eye, going to the posterior pole, and filling the eye in a posterior-to-anterior direction.[115]

After the vitreous cavity is filled with silicone oil, the needle used to inject silicone is removed along with the air infusion cannula, and the sclerotomies are sutured securely.

Injection of silicone into the vitreous cavity is invariably accompanied by the escape of a small amount of oil outside the eye. Frequently, a mixture of silicone (which is hydrophobic) and water forms over the corneal surface, under the infusion contact lens, interfering considerably with visibility. Bartov et al,[126] using methylcellulose 1.75% for contact lenses in 20 eyes undergoing silicone oil injection, found no difficulty with visualization. The investigators postulate the high viscosity of methylcellulose 1.75% prevented mixing with silicone oil. Methylcellulose was placed in a 10-mL syringe attached to the infusion contact lens and was injected in small increments by a scrub nurse when needed.

When a cataract is removed at the time of vitrectomy, the anterior or posterior capsule may be preserved, depending on the surgical technique. An intact anterior or posterior lens capsule prevents the displacement of the silicone oil from the vitreous cavity to the anterior chamber. This method decreases the postoperative complications, such as glaucoma and keratopathy, most frequently seen in aphakic patients who have received intravitreal silicone oil.[87,125]

An inferior peripheral iridectomy is performed to decrease the possibility of pupillary block glaucoma.[125] This iridectomy is only required in aphakic eyes. Because silicone oil floats in an aqueous medium, a superior peripheral iridectomy could be blocked by the oil. In a group of 88 aphakic eyes, after vitrectomy and fluid–silicone exchange, anterior segment complications were diminished in silicone-filled aphakic eyes with an inferior rather than a superior iridectomy. After a 6-month follow-up in eyes with a patent inferior iridectomy, no silicone was found in the anterior chamber, but there was a 50% incidence in eyes with a superior peripheral iridectomy.[88,90]

Using these techniques, the aphakic eye can be filled with silicone. Adequate expansion of the globe is maintained with the air pump system after an air–fluid exchange. The air pump system allows us to perform the air–silicone exchange in one procedure. Then silicone oil is injected under pressure into an eye that is already expanded by air. If the eye wall is allowed to collapse during the air–silicone exchange, the exchange will not be complete, and retinal folds may occur. However, care should be taken not to fill the anterior chamber with oil. This procedure also affords excellent monitoring of IOP during the surgical procedure.[110] In phakic and

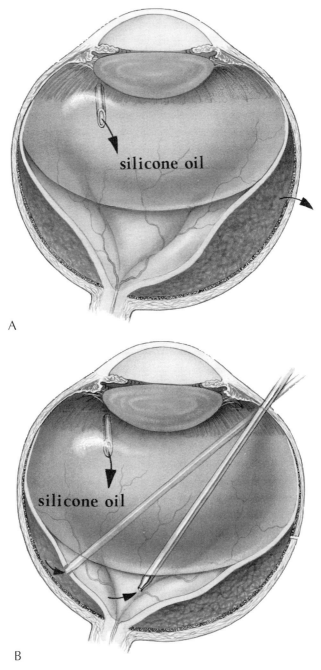

A

B

Figure 1–13. Graphic representation of the technique of silicone oil injection. **A.** While silicone oil is injected, subretinal fluid is simultaneously drained through a sclerotomy. **B.** Alternatively, silicone oil may be injected through a cannula while subretinal fluid is drained through a fluted needle.

pseudophakic eyes, the silicone bubble is allowed to just touch the posterior lens surface,[127] unless a cushion of vitreous separates the lens from the silicone bubble.

The second method of injection of silicone involves silicone–fluid exchange. When a silicone–fluid exchange is performed after vitrectomy, silicone is injected through the infusion line manually with a syringe or an automated pump while a fluted needle or extrusion handpiece with a silicone tube extending from the tip of the needle is used to drain subretinal fluid through a hole or drainage retinotomy (Fig. 1–13A, B). This procedure is followed by removal of preretinal fluid and then the fluid remaining inside the vitreous cavity.[128] Residual retinal traction detected during silicone injection can be relieved by a variety of vitreoretinal surgical techniques.[108,121]

Supplementary intravitreal injection of silicone may be required postoperatively in some eyes to achieve a complete fill of the vitreous cavity and to provide an adequate internal tamponade of all retinal tears. Further drainage of subretinal fluid that has reaccumulated, combined with an additional silicone injection, may be necessary to flatten the retina.[81,129]

SILICONE OIL REMOVAL FROM THE EYE

Vision-threatening complications resulting from intraocular silicone include cataract formation, elevated IOP, and corneal clouding.[30,60] In addition, diplopic symptoms related to the mirror effect of a silicone–aqueous interface (optical density approximately 1.4 and 1.0, respectively) have been reported.[30]

To avoid these problems, some investigators have recommended routine removal of liquid silicone from the eye after successful retinal reattachment.[98] When such complications are already present, silicone removal may be therapeutic.

Several techniques have been devised to remove intraocular silicone (Fig. 1–14).[76,99,108,130,131] A small temporal limbal incision can be made in aphakic eyes, whereas in phakic eyes a temporal superior sclerotomy is created and kept open with an iris spatula. A 21-gauge butterfly needle or a second infusion cannula connected to infusion fluid is placed through the inferior temporal pars plana into the midvitreous cavity. Silicone is lighter and floats on water. When the infusion fluid is allowed to flow inside the eye, silicone oil is expelled through the temporal opening.[76,108,130] However, small intraocular silicone bubbles may remain postoperatively.[76]

For patients with intracapsular aphakia, a modification of the technique is required. Air is injected into the anterior chamber, which pushes the silicone posteriorly beyond the iris plane. The globe is then rotated inferonasally (to bring the drainage sclerotomy superiormost), and a cotton-tipped applicator is used to apply pressure behind the limbus to help force silicone through the open sclerotomy. An alternative would be to create a limbal opening for silicone drainage instead of a pars plana sclerotomy.

The sclerotomies then are closed, the traction sutures are removed, and the conjunctiva is reapproximated in a routine manner. Subconjunctival injection of antibiotic and steroid completes the procedure.[131]

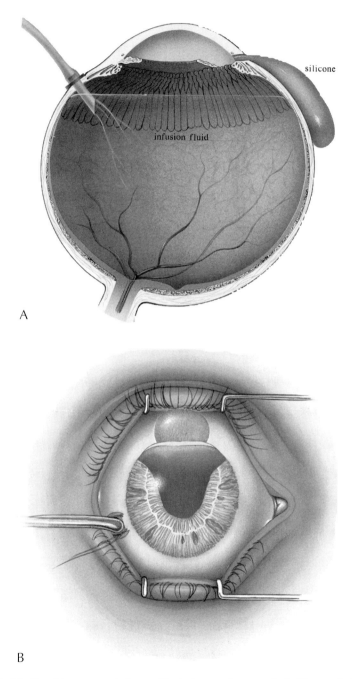

Figure 1–14. Graphic representations of techniques of removal of silicone. **A.** In aphakic eye. **B.** Front view. **C.** In phakic eye.

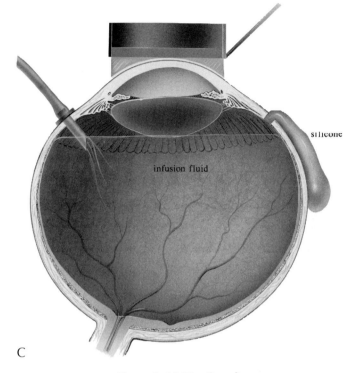

silicone

infusion fluid

C

Figure 1–14 (Continued).

MANAGEMENT OF SUBRETINAL SILICONE

If silicone oil has gained access to the subretinal space, a similar maneuver may be used for its removal. Initially, an anterior retinotomy is performed, and then the vitreous cavity is filled either with infusion fluid or with perfluorocarbon liquid. These substances force the subretinal silicone out of a superior retinotomy (Fig. 1–15).

SPECIFIC USES OF SILICONE OIL

Silicone Oil Techniques for Giant Retinal Tear

In contrast to gas, silicone provides a long-acting internal tamponade after repair of giant retinal tears; therefore, it may be preferable to gas, because of the high incidence of PVR after giant tear repair.[132-134]

A lensectomy may be performed when necessary to facilitate removal of vitreous in the region of the vitreous base, to allow dissection of preretinal membranes in eyes with anterior PVR, and to improve visualization in eyes with significant lenticular opacities.[135]

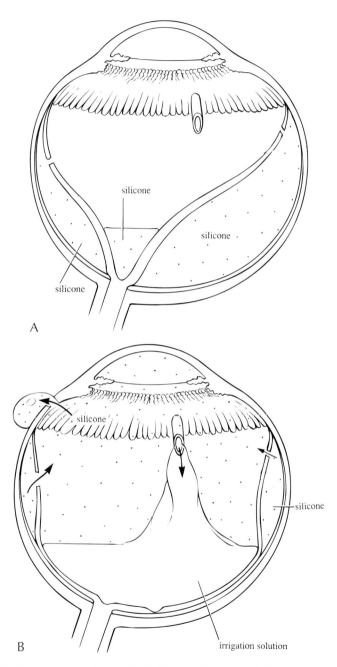

Figure 1–15. Management of subretinal silicone oil. **A.** A peripheral retinotomy is performed. **B.** Irrigating solution is injected into the vitreous cavity, forcing subretinal silicone out of the vitreous cavity through the retinotomy.

Using scleral indentations, vitreous is removed as completely as possible from the region of the vitreous base and ciliary body.[71,132,133,136,137] Visualization may be improved with coaxial illumination.[135]

After completion of the vitrectomy, the posterior edge of the giant tear is grasped with a forceps or with the silicone-tipped back-flush brush needle. The retina is gently elevated and the eye rotated so that the tear is held in a dependent position.[133]

When manual attempts to maintain the retina in the proper anatomic position are impossible, a variety of mechanical fixation techniques are available.[71,132]

At this point, silicone oil is injected through an infusion cannula. While a fluid–silicone exchange is performed, the posteriorly located fluid is evacuated from the retinal surface.[132,133,138]

When a giant tear is complicated by PVR, the detached retina may be almost totally immobile.[71,132-134,136,137] The eye is rotated so that the giant tear is in a dependent position, and silicone oil is injected intravitreally. The torn edge of the retina must be held against the retinal pigment epithelium until silicone reaches the retina. Silicone injection is then continued, with preretinal and subretinal fluid evacuated.

After retinal reattachment, endophotocoagulation or argon laser photocoagulation may be applied in two to three nonconfluent rows near the posterior margin of the giant tear or in a single confluent row using an indirect ophthalmoscope delivery system.[132-134,137]

An encircling scleral buckle is placed at the end of the procedure. The sclerotomies are left open to allow silicone oil to leave the eye when the buckle is tightened. The buckle should include the vitreous base and the ends of the giant tear.[132,133,137]

Billington and Leaver[136] reviewed a series of eyes with giant retinal tears treated with vitrectomy and fluid–silicone oil exchange. The retina remained reattached in 63 of 73 eyes (86%) at 6 months after surgery and in 54 of 65 eyes (83%) 18 months after surgery. Eight patients were lost to follow-up between the 6- and 18-month examinations.

Silicone Oil Use in PVR

A number of factors have increased the success rate of surgical management of eyes previously considered to be either unsalvageable or to have an extremely poor prognosis because of retinal detachments complicated by severe PVR. These include an improved understanding of the pathophysiology of PVR and new vitreoretinal microsurgical techniques. Other improvements include the use of different intravitreal substances to reposition the retina and tamponade retinal breaks and the development of recent technologic advances in equipment.[60,71,101,103,114,123,129,139-151]

Aaberg[152] presented his results in managing 98 consecutive cases of nontraumatic nondiabetic PVR (grades C_3 through D_3) from January 1983 through June 1987. Eighty of these eyes were followed for an additional 6 months after surgery. Intraocular tamponade was provided by gas or silicone, with relaxing retinotomies performed in 14 eyes. Thirty-three eyes demonstrated only posterior PVR. Seventy percent of eyes within this group, which were followed for an average period of 11 months, had completely attached retinas, and an additional 12% demonstrated retinal attachment just posterior to the buckle, which gave a total reattachment rate of 82%. In contrast, only 57% (27 of 47 eyes) with a significant anterior component achieved total retinal attachment. An additional 10 eyes in this group demonstrated an attached retina just posterior to the buckle, which gave a 79% overall reattachment rate for these eyes.

Several authors had reported encouraging results indicating a high success rate in the treatment of complicated retinal detachment with vitrectomy techniques and silicone oil.[25,34,76,88,99,102,142,143,153-158] However, the functional success rate is not as great as the anatomic success.[142,143,158] The rate of success was reported to range from 27% to 77%, depending on the time of the evaluation after silicone injection. The anatomic success (70%) is better than the functional success (60%) in a series of 500 cases with a 2-year follow-up reported by Lucke et al.[142] A similar observation was noted by Yeo et al in 1987.[143] This finding can be explained by the fact that retinal detachment has a very poor prognosis.

Fluid–silicone exchange is preferred by some surgeons for the following situations: (1) suspected or "lost" retinal breaks obscured by preretinal hemorrhage; (2) posterior retinal breaks, especially if not treated with intraoperative photocoagulation or cryopexy; (3) persistent tangential traction associated with retinal breaks; (4) multiple retinal breaks, particularly when widely separated; and (5) eyes requiring permanent intraocular tamponade because of tightly adherent and permanently contracted epiretinal membranes (ERMs) that require retinal resection to relieve traction.[159]

The amount of silicone oil injected to fill the vitreous cavity differs from one eye to another. Usually complete vitrectomy is followed by fluid–air exchange (Figs. 1–16), with the injection of 3 to 4 mL of silicone oil.[153] Other investigators report a similar technique.[143] To avoid glaucoma and keratopathy, and to allow the aqueous the opportunity to circulate, we do not fill the eye completely. We initially position the patient face-down so that the silicone will tamponade the retina and prevent inferior accumulation of fluid.

Silicone oil is usually removed from the eye when the retina is attached, chorioretinal scars are formed, and there is no traction in the retina. McCuen et al[76] suggested removal 3 to 6 months after intravitreal injection. A similar suggestion was made by Sell et al.[144] Lucke et al,[142] in their series of 500 patients, removed silicone oil in periods ranging between 6 and 18 months, with an average of 9.5 months. Federman and Schubert[38] removed silicone oil in their series between 3 and 30 months after intraocular injection. Gonvers[108] removes silicone oil 6 to 8 weeks after vitrectomy; he suggests that this interval allows adequate time for chorioretinal adhesions to become firm while the proliferative process becomes quiet.

Repair of recurrent inferior retinal detachments under silicone oil requires repeated membrane peeling and, occasionally, a relaxing retinotomy. When the detachment is the result of an open retinal break in the absence of a contributing tractional component, the redetachment is caused by the inadequate tamponading effect of silicone. Scott[155] advocates injecting additional silicone to correct this situation,

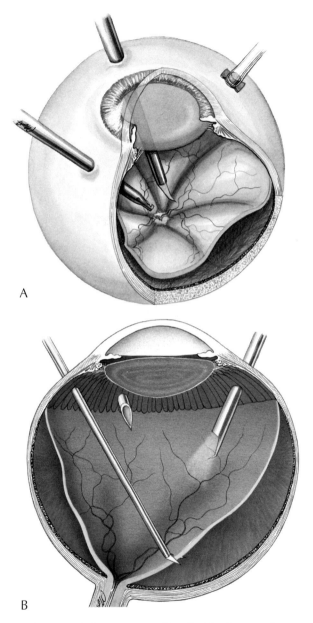

A

B

Figure 1–16. Technique of vitrectomy combined with silicone oil injection in posterior PVR. **A.** After removal of anterior and posterior PVR using membrane pick and scissors. **B.** A hole is created for drainage of the subretinal fluid.

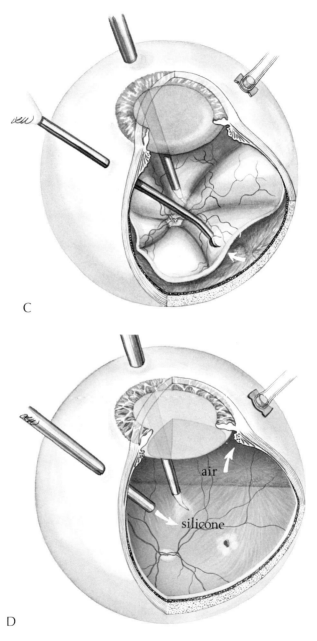

C

D

Figure 1–16 (Continued). C. Internal drainage of subretinal fluid is carried out. **D.** After a complete air–fluid exchange, the air is replaced with silicone.

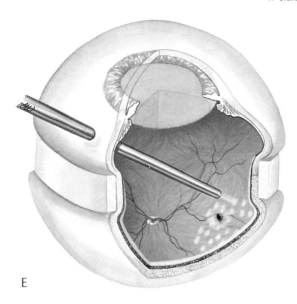

E

Figure 1–16 (Continued). E.   Photocoagulation of the retina is performed with endolaser under the silicone.

whereas Sternberg and Meredith[160] recommend positioning the patient face-down. This position allows the silicone bubble to tamponade the hole by remaining in apposition with the inferior retina. Additional photocoagulation is performed when the retina flattens.

In phakic and pseudophakic eyes, the likelihood of silicone oil entering the anterior chamber is small.[38,91,151,161] Riedel and associates[151] postulated that silicone is able to reach the anterior chamber by passing around either the crystalline or intraocular lens. This movement is made possible by partial zonulysis occurring during extracapsular cataract extraction or as a result of trauma. In other eyes, the high IOP present during air–fluid exchange or intraocular silicone oil injection appears to create partial zonulysis. In a series of 415 patients[151] treated with silicone oil with a viscosity of 5,000 cSt, these investigators reported the presence of silicone oil in the anterior chambers of 6% of their phakic and pseudophakic patients. Silicone oil was more frequently present in the anterior chamber of these eyes after direct injection, in contrast to administration after air–fluid exchange. The postoperative use of miotics may prevent silicone oil from reentering the anterior chamber in some eyes.

Causes of silicone penetration into the anterior chamber in aphakia include high IOP, an incomplete iris diaphragm, overfilling of the eye with silicone oil, and loss of patency of the inferior iridectomy. When the pupil is not extremely dilated, and good view of the iris is not obstructed, an inferior iridectomy that has been closed off by fibrinous membranes can be opened using Nd:YAG laser. Alternatively, surgery may be used to reopen the iridectomies. Protrusion of silicone oil in the anterior chamber may be avoided when (1) surgery is completed with the eye at near-normal IOP; (2) overfilling with silicone oil is avoided; (3) recurrent retinal detachment is prevented, which causes a decrease in the volume of the vitreous cavity and is associated with silicone oil in the anterior chamber; (4) large superior iridectomy is avoided so that the iris diaphragm is retained.[79]

In phakic eyes, silicone in the anterior chamber can be removed by making two stab incisions 180° apart at the limbus. A small cannula placed through the smaller incision is used to inject infusion fluid or Healon, which gradually pushes silicone out of the larger incision. After removal of all the silicone from the anterior chamber, the larger incision is closed with 9–0 nylon suture, and the Healon is irrigated away.[162]

To avoid overfill, some of the silicone oil can be removed through a sclerotomy if deemed appropriate, and an elevated IOP is avoided at the end of intravitreal injection. Additionally, both during and at the termination of fluid–silicone exchange or air–silicone exchange, either fluid or air is kept in the anterior chamber.[76]

When a direct silicone–fluid exchange is performed, removal of silicone oil that has inadvertently entered the anterior chamber of aphakic eyes during injection should be delayed until the vitreous cavity is almost completely filled with silicone oil. A cannula inserted through the pars plana into the anterior chamber is used to inject a viscoelastic material, which forces the silicone posteriorly behind the iris diaphragm.[163]

In aphakic eyes with an intact iris diaphragm, silicone oil can block the superior iridectomy and cause pupillary block. Aqueous accumulating at the 6-o'clock position behind the iris diaphragm may force silicone oil into the anterior chamber. Even with the patient in a prone position, once silicone has entered the anterior chamber, the inability of aqueous to pass from the posterior to anterior chamber prevents silicone oil from returning to the vitreous cavity. An iridectomy at the 6-clock-hour position wide enough to avoid obstruction by the inflammatory reaction should prevent pupillary block. An iridectomy can be performed routinely using a vitrectomy instrument at the end of vitrectomy in aphakic eyes before intraocular injection of silicone oil (Fig. 1–8), or using an Nd:YAG laser after injection of silicone oil.

Beekhuis and associates[163] gently aspirate the basal iris into the port of the suction cutter and then activate the cutting mode until a hole at least 2 mm in diameter is created. When a lensectomy becomes necessary in an eye previously filled with silicone, an inferior surgical iridectomy or laser iridectomy can be performed before removal of the cataract.[88,163]

Accumulation of silicone oil in the anterior chamber of an aphakic eye despite a patent basal iridectomy at 6 o'clock has three causes: an inadequately sized iridectomy; low aqueous production, insufficient to circulate into the anterior chamber in eyes that have undergone multiple procedures; or a tractional retinal detachment, which can cause a volume reduction in the vitreous cavity.[163]

However, Elliott et al[164] found that a superior iridectomy might be effective in preventing pupillary block caused by silicone oil in patients who had previously undergone vitrectomy with intravitreal silicone injection followed by intracapsular cataract extraction as a second procedure. Whether a superior iridectomy will be as effective as an inferior iridectomy in preventing pupillary block injection is not known because a comparative study was not performed.[164]

Silicone Oil versus Gas in PVR

The Silicone Study Group[97] conducted a multicenter, randomized clinical trial involving 101 eyes with rhegmatogenous retinal detachment and severe PVR (grade C_3 or worse) to compare the effectiveness of silicone oil and SF_6 as tamponading agents. Eyes without prior vitrectomy (group I) were vitrectomized and treated with either a mixture of 20% SF_6 and air or 1,000-cSt silicone oil. Follow-up extended up to 36 months in most cases. Fifty percent to sixty percent of eyes treated with silicone oil showed visual acuity of 5/200 or better as compared with 30% to 40% of those treated with SF_6. The silicone oil–treated eyes also showed more frequent macular attachment (80% versus 60%). Macular detachment was more prevalent in eyes with hypotony (40% to 50% for SF_6, 25% to 30% for silicone oil) and keratopathy (55% to 60%). This study indicates that silicone oil is superior to SF_6 gas in the treatment of PVR.

In another multicenter, randomized study, the Silicone Study Group[106] treated 265 eyes with rhegmatogenous retinal detachment and severe PVR (grade C_3 or worse) and compared the effectiveness of silicone oil and perfluoropropane gas (C_3F_8) as tamponading agents. Prior vitrectomy had not been performed on 131 of these eyes (group I); 134 had undergone prior vitrectomy with intraocular gas tamponade (group II). Both groups underwent vitrectomy and were treated with either 14% C_3F_8 and air or silicone oil (1,000 cSt). Follow-up ranged up to 36 months. At final examination, no significant difference was found between eyes treated with silicone oil and those treated with C_3F_8 in achievement of visual acuity greater than or equal to 5/200 or retinal reattachment. Complete posterior retinal reattachment was achieved more often in eyes without prior vitrectomy (group I) that received C_3F_8. Hypotony was twice as prevalent in eyes that received C_3F_8 and was more common in eyes that had prior vitrectomy (group II) tamponaded with that gas. Although the first study[97] demonstrated that, in the treatment of PVR, silicone is a better tamponading agent than SF_6, the second report[106] indicated little difference between silicone oil and C_3F_8 gas.[105]

Silicone Study Report 3[165] found no significant differences present between eyes in both groups during final follow-up examination regarding macular reattachment (78% versus 77%), visual acuity of 5/200 or better (44% versus 36%), or complete retinal detachment posterior to the encircling scleral buckle. Comparing outcome between group I and group II eyes, there was no difference in hypotony (IOP of 5 mm Hg or less) or persistent elevation of IOP to 30 mm Hg or more, but a higher frequency of keratopathy in group II eyes.

The investigators suggested that the increased number of vitrectomies, along with the greater amount of aphakic eyes when comparing eyes in group II with those in group I, were the factors responsible for the increased frequency of keratopathy reported in group II. The likelihood of eyes achieving a visual acuity of 5/200 or better was greater in eyes in which retinal reattachment was achieved after a single procedure (66%) in contrast to eyes requiring multiple operations (45%).[165]

Follow-up data in the report were available for 97% of group I eyes at 6 months and 60% of group I at 36 months versus 99% of group II after 6 months and 56% of group II eyes after 36 months.

Results of the Silicone Study[166] suggest that retinotomy is required more frequently in eyes requiring additional vitreoretinal surgery for PVR where silicone oil and perfluorocarbon gases were equally effective tamponading agents. In contrast, silicone oil and perfluorocarbon gas were equally effective tamponading agents in group II eyes requiring retinotomy.

Retinotomy was performed more than twice as frequently in group II (41%) than in group I eyes (20%).[166] At the 6-month postoperative examination, visual acuity or retinal status of eyes undergoing retinotomy in group I but not group II with a silicone oil tamponade had a lower incidence of hypotony and better anatomic results. From 6 to 24 months, a trend toward improvement was noted in the perfluorocarbon-filled eyes, whereas worsening was noted in the silicone-filled eyes.[166]

We compared the effects of intravitreal silicone oil with those of long-lasting gas (C_3F_8 or C_4F_8) in the management of complicated retinal detachment and vitreous hemorrhage.[153] The randomization was stratified into four diagnostic categories, so that the factors influencing each condition could be properly analyzed. Although we recruited different numbers of patients in each category, a similar-to-equal number of patients between treatment groups was sustained. Moreover, the even distribution of the patients for age and sex, preoperative vitreoretinal status, and severity of PVR demonstrated that the randomization provided fairly matched treatment groups.

The overall rate of reattachment was 82% for the oil-treated group and 83% for the gas-treated group. The visual acuity was unchanged or improved in 72% of the oil-treated and 76% of the gas-treated patients, demonstrating a similar response to each treatment during the follow-up period of this study. The similar anatomic and visual results between treatment groups were demonstrated in the categories of proliferative diabetic retinopathy with retinal detachment, PVR, and traumatic retinal detachment. Although this result could be attributed to the small sample size, the consistent pattern of equal treatment outcome under our surgical procedure may have been the result of a minimum true difference in effectiveness between the two treatment groups. At least, we were confident (90%, 1-beta, power) that the difference between the two treatment outcomes was less than 40% effectiveness from this sample size (alpha = .1. N = 50. beta = .1. difference of effectiveness = .31 ~ .36).

We had recruited most study subjects with moderately severe complicated retinal detachment or vitreous hemorrhage in terms of operability, which presumably was inversely related to the number of previously failed surgeries. Those with inoperable retinal detachments and simple, early stages of retinal detachment were excluded in the entry criteria to prevent masking of the difference between the two treatment outcomes. However, the grading of PVR in the categories of PVR and traumatic retinal detachment indicated fewer cases of PVR D_{1-3}, particularly D_3 stage in the traumatic category. This may have been attributable to the small sampling or the uneven distribution of the underlying population. Nevertheless, this limited our results as applied to those cases.

Despite the similar outcomes between the treatment groups, we observed significant differences in the occurrence of postoperative complications. Late elevation of IOP occurred significantly more frequently (P = .009) in the gas-treated group than in the oil-treated group, partially as a result of repeated gas–fluid exchanges in the former.

Postoperative vitreous hemorrhage occurred more commonly in the gas-treated eyes than in the oil-treated eyes (P = .045). This discovery supported our speculation that silicone oil in the vitreous cavity may have helped to prevent vitreous hemorrhage or may have kept the bleeding localized to a small area. In the category of proliferative diabetic retinopathy with vitreous hemorrhage without retinal detachment, which was initially chosen to gauge the prevention of rubeosis iridis and the decrease in postoperative vitreous hemorrhage with the use of intravitreal silicone oil, all cases receiving oil succeeded without recurrent vitreous hemorrhage, and the case receiving gas had recurrent vitreous hemorrhage postoperatively. The effect of silicone oil on the prevention of vitreous hemorrhage and the outcome after the removal of silicone oil, particularly in cases of proliferative diabetic retinopathy, necessitates further investigations.

Localized retinal detachments occurred more often in gas-treated than in oil-treated eyes (P < .25). Reabsorption of the gas from the vitreous cavity and the subsequent decrease in retinal tamponade may have contributed to this complication. Because localized peripheral retinal detachments in the gas-treated group were managed with fluid–gas exchanges and argon laser photocoagulation, the oil-treated eyes required fewer procedures to achieve a stable condition.

In the category of proliferative diabetic retinopathy with retinal detachment, visual acuity was not improved in approximately half the patients in each treatment group in spite of the good anatomic success rate (80%). The poor visual acuity in some cases without macular lesions may be explained by capillary dropout in the macular area and optic nerve atrophy commonly seen in end-stage diabetic disease.

Although we had speculated that silicone might reduce the risk of postoperative rubeosis, two patients (20%) in our oil-treated group developed rubeosis iridis postoperatively. We believe that factors such as aphakia and the presence or absence of retinal detachment may have played a more important role in the occurrence of rubeosis than the presence of intravitreal silicone oil.

One eye in the silicone oil-treated group that was considered an anatomic failure underwent removal of the oil, preretinal membrane peeling, and intravitreal gas injection with subsequent anatomic success. Similarly, one eye in the gas-treated group with a redetached retina was treated with intravitreal silicone injection and achieved attachment. These cases demonstrated that repeated procedures with similar or different techniques may be necessary to achieve success in complicated cases.

We observed further progression of PVR that resulted in anatomic failure in two cases of PVR and traumatic retinal detachment that were treated with intravitreal silicone oil. This indicated that the oil does not prevent the progression or development of preretinal membranes and that the therapeutic value of silicone oil is in the mechanical tamponading of the retina and not in the inhibition of cell proliferation.

We used 12,500-cSt silicone oil in our study. The amount of silicone oil injected intravitreally correlated well with the occurrence of postoperative retinal detachment. When the intravitreal silicone oil volume was less than 3.0 mL, detachment was more frequent (P = .03). We believe that the amount of silicone oil injected should range from 3.0 to 5.0 mL. Higher volumes may produce increased IOP. Further studies are needed to clarify this factor.

The efficacy of the two intravitreal gases used could not be assessed, because patients were not randomized to either one. The C_3F_8 lasted longer in the vitreous cavity than the C_4F_8 and may have decreased the need for subsequent fluid–gas exchanges. In this study, we used an air–gas mixture to minimize complications associated with pure intravitreal gas. It is possible that a different result may be achieved in a randomized trial with pure gas as compared with silicone oil. However, this hypothesis requires further investigation.

In conclusion, we believe that both silicone oil and long-lasting gases are important tools in the management of complicated retinal detachment and vitreous hemorrhage. The use of one or the other should be at the discretion of the surgeon experienced in their application. Despite the limited sample size, this randomized study demonstrated the short-term value of each method and the significant difference in the postoperative occurrence of complications in the two treatment modalities. However, in this preliminary study, silicone oil was left in the eye except when it produced complications. Further follow-up is needed for evaluation of long-term complications of intravitreal silicone oil.

Silicone Oil as an Intravitreal Drug Delivery Vehicle

Silicone oil has been tested as a repository for lipophilic antiproliferative agents.[167-169] In vivo models of PVR have responded. In vivo data demonstrated retinoic acid,[167] retinol,[168] and carmustine (BCNU)[169] dissolved in silicone oil were effective in the treatment of PVR in rabbit eyes. These experiments suggest that in the future silicone oil also may have a role as an intravitreal drug delivery vehicle in eyes with PVR when this substance is used as an internal tamponading agent.[167-169]

Use of Silicone Oil in Diabetic Vitrectomy

Silicone oil usually has been reserved for diabetic eyes with minimal or no prospect of a successful result after conventional vitrectomy surgery. These indications have included: (1) eyes with severe tractional retinal detachment, possibly requiring a retinotomy or retinectomy to relieve residual traction;[170] (2) failed vitrectomy surgery in eyes with a rhegmatogenous retinal detachment that develop PVR;[171] (3) recurrent, nonclearing vitreous hemorrhage, where injection of silicone oil will keep the vitreous cavity clear by preventing rebleeding, allowing the subsequent use of laser;[170] (4) rubeosis irides associated with complications of proliferative diabetic retinopathy.[172]

Diabetes mellitus is a major cause of rubeosis iridis.[172] The incidence of preoperative rubeosis in diabetic eyes[173] has been reported to be approximately 13%.[174] The incidence of rubeosis iridis after lensectomy and vitrectomy ranges from 30% to 50%.[175-177] When only vitrectomy is performed, the incidence of rubeosis iridis has been 10% to 15%.[178]

Silicone has been postulated by some investigators to prevent or arrest the development of rubeosis irides,[170,172] whereas other investigators have questioned this benefit.[127,171,174] In one large series[170] involving 106 diabetic eyes treated with vitrectomy and silicone oil injection, 26% of eyes had rubeosis preoperatively. Subsequently, rubeosis disappeared in 13 of these eyes and progressed in only three.

New rubeosis occurred in 13% of the cases but demonstrated no correlation with the risk factors of aphakia or retinal detachment. Animal experiments have demonstrated that the anterior chamber oxygen concentration is higher in aphakic vitrectomized eyes with silicone injection than in similar eyes not filled with silicone.[177] This effect has been attributed to a barrier effect caused by silicone. Silicone may prevent the uptake of oxygen by the retina, which is considerably less oxygenated than the circulating aqueous humor. Similarly, a neovascular factor elaborated by detached retina may be prevented in various degrees from reaching the anterior segment, depending on the completeness of the silicone fill of the vitreous and preretinal space. In the presence of a complete fill, forward diffusion of this substance may be prevented, causing regression or preventing development of rubeosis irides.[159,170,179,180] Additionally, in eyes with rubeosis irides, silicone oil injection is often accompanied by retinal reattachment, which may eliminate the stimulus for iris neovascularization.[170]

Azzolini et al[181] demonstrated that aphakic vitrectomized eyes, despite the presence of a silicone oil tamponade, have a higher risk of developing iris diabetic microangiopathy. The study also demonstrated that marked anterior segment postoperative inflammation is a risk factor for worsening of diabetic microangiopathy.

Rinkoff and associates[171] concluded that silicone oil did not prevent the development of anterior segment neovascularization but lessened the likelihood of intractable elevated IOP in these eyes. Brourman et al[179] found similar results. After the use of silicone oil for treatment of severe proliferative diabetic retinopathy, regression of rubeosis irides occurred in only 8 of 22 eyes.

McCuen et al[182] performed revision vitrectomy with silicone injection in 18 diabetic eyes. These eyes had severe anterior ocular neovascularization, progressive iris neovascularization, or anterior hyaloidal fibrovascular proliferation complicated by severe retinal detachment with C_3–C_4 PVR or media opacity. In five eyes, there was regression, and in 10 eyes, there was no increase in anterior segment neovascularization. The rest demonstrated further progression of these changes postoperatively. Three eyes were treated with endolaser to the ciliary processes to control IOP, and no eyes in this series developed persistent uncontrolled postoperative IOP increases.

Reproliferation originating from isolated membrane epicenters that have not been surgically removed may occur, causing tractional retinal detachments.[127,170] Silicone appears to provide a space for tissue growth and may concentrate growth factors and fibrin, stimulating replication.[170,183] To eliminate or reduce this reproliferation, the epicenters can be removed during surgery with retinotomies and more extensive membrane dissection.[170,183]

Wilson-Holt and Gregor[184] described the spontaneous relief of inferior tractional retinal detachments by large peripheral tension tears that coalesced into relaxing retinotomies in six diabetic eyes after vitrectomy with silicone oil tamponade. These eyes had a minimum follow-up period of 12 months. The epiretinal proliferation responsible for these events occurred 2 to 4 months after vitrectomy. The posterior retina remained attached in all eyes because the process was limited to the anterior retina.

Silicone oil maintains both a prolonged and stable internal tamponade[12] in eyes having preexisting retinal holes or iatrogenic tears. This factor may minimize problems associated with retinal tears caused by membrane peeling.[99,142,179] In contrast to gas, no special postoperative positioning is necessary. Because of the optical clarity of silicone, hemostatic effects, and minimal refractive changes, visual rehabilitation is quicker. Fundus details are more clearly visible through silicone than through gas, thus facilitating both the intraoperative and postoperative use of laser photocoagulation in silicone-filled diabetic eyes.[142,179]

Silicone oil tamponade may be indicated in eyes in which preretinal hemorrhage, subretinal hemorrhage, or a residual layer of subretinal fluid prevents intraoperative laser treatment of retinal tears or a retinotomy at the time of surgery.[185] Silicone oil, in contrast to gas, provides a more permanent retinal tamponade and permits excellent retinal visualization. These properties permit the surgeon to wait several weeks if necessary until the blood or subretinal fluid is reabsorbed. At this time, placement of laser photocoagulation is possible to seal the retinal tears or a retinotomy, which is mandatory if permanent retinal reattachment is to be achieved.

Redetachment after vitrectomy may occur from an open hole or reproliferation. The mechanical effects of a silicone-filled eye limit the extent and rapidity of the detachment, often resulting in the macula remaining attached for long periods and usually allowing necessary surgery to be performed at a convenient time.

Lucke and associates[142] used silicone oil after pars plana vitrectomy in 106 eyes with proliferative diabetic retinopathy. Silicone oil was used to tamponade large or multiple posterior retinal tears and to prevent recurrent postoperative vitreous hemorrhage in 90 eyes with retinal detachment. Usually these eyes had combined rhegmatogenous and tractional components and florid PVR. Sixteen eyes received intraocular silicone for hemostatic reasons, despite an attached retina. After 24 months, anatomic attachment existed in 65% of the eyes. Ambulatory vision was achieved in 48% of eyes at this postoperative interval. Results were much better in the eyes in which the retina was attached preoperatively, and silicone was used for hemostatic reasons.

Rinkoff and associates[171] reported results in 10 diabetic eyes with retinal detachment complicated by PVR after vitrectomy with intraocular silicone injection. Postoperative retinal reattachment was achieved in all 10 eyes. After a minimum follow-up of 1 year, a total retinal detachment was seen in three eyes. Intraocular pressure was low to normal in nine eyes.

Recurrent vitreous hemorrhage sufficient to obscure details of the posterior pole was present in one series in 16% of phakic patients and 21% of aphakic patients 6 months after vitrectomy.[186] Silicone oil prevents recurrent vitreous hemorrhage, providing a clear intraocular media postoperatively. The use of silicone oil in cases of nonclearing vitreous hemorrhage is limited by the availability of other methods of removing intraocular blood and achieving retinal tamponade. Monocular patients with a limited life expectancy and recurrent or persistent vitreous hemorrhage are one group of patients who may benefit from silicone injection.[170]

Pearson and associates[187] evaluated the outcome after removal of silicone oil in 25 diabetic eyes that had undergone successful vitrectomy with retinal reattachment for complicated retinal detachments associated with proliferative diabetic retinopathy. The retina was reattached after surgery in all eyes.

Pearson and associates noted that the 12% incidence (3 of 25 eyes) of retinal detachment after silicone oil removal was lower than that reported for nondiabetics.[74,76,99] The investigators suggested that pathophysiologic differences between diabetic and nondiabetic eyes may in part explain this difference in rate of retinal detachment after silicone oil removal. The investigators noted that iatrogenic or pre-existing retinal breaks are usually preequatorial in the diabetic patient, because the proliferative process is generally limited to this area. The posterior location makes these retinal breaks very accessible when any associated traction must be relieved. In contrast, retinal tears in eyes with PVR, especially when complicated by anterior PVR, tend to be located in peripheral retina, which makes permanent closure more difficult.

Additionally, scatter laser photocoagulation applied to eyes in this series[187] strengthened retinal adhesions, lessening the likelihood of retinal detachment after silicone oil removal.

REFERENCES

1. Crisp A, de Juan E Jr, Tiedeman J: Effect of silicone oil viscosity on emulsification. *Arch Ophthalmol* 1987;105:546–550.
2. Gabel VP, Kampik A, Burkhart J: Analysis of intraocularly applied silicone oils of various origins. *Graefes Arch Clin Exp Ophthalmol* 1987;225:160–162.
3. Hammer ME, Rinder DF, Hicks EL, et al: Tolerance of perfluorocarbons, fluorosilicone, and silicone liquids in the vitreous, in Freeman HM, Tolentino FI (eds): *Proliferative Vitreoretinopathy (PVR)*. New York: Springer-Verlag, 1988, pp 156–161.
4. Pon DM: Chemical characteristics of perfluorocarbon liquids and silicone oil for complex retinal detachments. *Vitreoretinal Surg Technol* 1990;2(1):6.
5. Živojnović R: *Silicone Oil in Vitreoretinal Surgery*. Dordrecht, The Netherlands: Martinus Nijhoff/Dr W Junk Pub, 1987, pp 40–44.
6. Wilson-Holt N, Leaver PK: Extended criteria for vitrectomy and fluid/silicone oil exchange. *Eye* 1990;4:850–854.
7. Kreiner CF: Chemical and physical aspects of clinically applied silicones. *Dev Ophthalmol* 1987;14:11–19.
8. Schepens CL: *Retinal Detachment and Allied Diseases*. Philadelphia: WB Saunders, 1983, p 749.
9. Cibis PA: Symposium: Present status of retinal detachment surgery: Vitreous transfer and silicone injections. *Trans Am Acad Ophthalmol Otolaryngol* 1964; 68:983–997.
10. Petersen J: The physical and surgical aspects of silicone in the vitreous cavity. *Graefes Arch Clin Exp Ophthalmol* 1987;225:452–456.
11. Yoshizumi MO, Dunn B, Ligh JK, et al: Physical properties of vitamin E oil and silicone oil. *Retina* 1985;5:163–167.
12. De Juan E Jr, McCuen B, Tiedeman J: Intraocular tamponade and surface tension. *Surv Ophthalmol* 1985;30:47–51.
13. Leaver PK: Long-standing retinal detachments: The role of internal tamponade. *Trans Ophthalmol Soc UK* 1986;105:476–479.

14. Haut J, Larricart JP, van Effenterre G, et al: Some of the most important properties of silicone oil to explain its action. *Ophthalmologica* 1985;191:150–153.
15. Smith RC, Smith GT, Wong D: Refractive changes in silicone filled eyes. *Eye* 1990;4:230–234.
16. Stone W Jr: Alloplasty in surgery of the eye. *N Engl J Med* 1958;258:486–490.
17. Cibis PA, Becker B, Okun E, et al: The use of liquid silicone in retinal detachment surgery. *Arch Ophthalmol* 1962;68:590–599.
18. Cibis PA: *Vitreoretinal Pathology and Surgery in Retinal Detachment.* St Louis: CV Mosby, 1965, pp 80, 92, 125, 133.
19. Cibis PA: Recent methods in the surgical treatment of retinal detachment: Intravitreal procedures. *Trans Ophthalmol Soc UK* 1965;85:111–127.
20. Armaly MF: Ocular tolerance to silicones: I. Replacement of aqueous and vitreous by silicone fluids. *Arch Ophthalmol* 1962;68:390–395.
21. Moreau PG: Implants into the vitreous using silicone for detachment of the retina. *Trans Ophthalmol Soc UK* 1964;84:167–171.
22. Niesel P, Fankhauser F: Zur retrovitrealen Silikoninjektion bei der Behandlung der Netzhautablösung. *Ophthalmologica* 1964;147:167–175.
23. Kanski JJ, Daniel R: Intravitreal silicone injection in retinal detachment. *Br J Ophthalmol* 1973;57:542–545.
24. Dufour R: Experience with intraocular silicone injection, in McPherson A (ed): *New and Controversial Aspects of Retinal Detachment.* New York: Harper & Row, 1968, pp 377–382.
25. Watzke RC: Silicone retinopiesis for retinal detachment: A long-term clinical evaluation. *Arch Ophthalmol* 1967;77:185–196.
26. Watzke RC: Silicone retinopiesis for retinal detachment: A pathologic report. *Surv Ophthalmol* 1967;12:333–337.
27. Cockerham W, Schepens CL, Freeman HM: Silicone injection in retinal detachment. *Mod Probl Ophthalmol* 1969;8:525–540.
28. Mukai N, Lee P-F, Oguri M, et al: A long-term evaluation of silicone retinopathy in monkeys. *Can J Ophthalmol* 1975;10:391–402.
29. Machemer R: Synopsis of Vail: Third Vitreous Seminar, March 8–15, 1980, Vail, CO. *Int Ophthalmol* 1980;2:175–177.
30. Haut J, Ullern M, Chermet M, et al: Complications of intraocular injections of silicone combined with vitrectomy. *Ophthalmologica* 1980;180:29–35.
31. Ober RR, Blanks JC, Ogden TE, et al: Experimental retinal tolerance to liquid silicone. *Retina* 1983;3:77–85.
32. Labelle P, Okun E: Ocular tolerance to liquid silicone: An experimental study. *Can J Ophthalmol* 1972;7:199–204.
33. Scott JD: A rationale for the use of liquid silicone in retinal detachment surgery, in Shimizu K, Oosterhuis JA (eds): *XXIII Concilium Ophthalmologicum, Kyoto, 1978, Acta.* Amsterdam: Excerpta Medica, 1979, pp 433–437.
34. Lean JS, Leaver PK, Cooling RJ, et al: Management of complex retinal detachments by vitrectomy and fluid/silicone exchange. *Trans Ophthalmol Soc UK* 1982; 102:203–205.
35. Grey RHB, Leaver PK: Results of silicone oil injection in massive preretinal retraction. *Trans Ophthalmol Soc UK* 1977;97:238–241.
36. Franks WA, Leaver PK: Removal of silicone oil: Rewards and penalties. *Eye* 1991;5:333–337.
37. Pang MP, Peyman GA, Kao GW: Early anterior segment complications after silicone oil injection. *Can J Ophthalmol* 1986;21:271–275.

38. Federman JL, Schubert HD: Complications associated with the use of silicone oil in 150 eyes after retina-vitreous surgery. *Ophthalmology* 1988;95:870–876.
39. Leaver PK: Silicone-oil injection in the treatment of massive preretinal retraction, in McPherson A (ed): *New and Controversial Aspects of Vitreoretinal Surgery*. St Louis: CV Mosby, 1977, pp 397–401.
40. Mukai N, Lee P-F, Schepens CL: Intravitreous injection of silicone: An experimental study: II. Histochemistry and electron microscopy. *Ann Ophthalmol* 1972;4:273–287.
41. Lee P-F, Donovan RH, Mukai N, et al: Intravitreous injection of silicone: An experimental study: I. Clinical picture and histology of the eye. *Ann Ophthalmol* 1969;1(2):15–25.
42. Ni C, Wang W-J, Albert DM, et al: Intravitreous silicone injection: Histopathologic findings in a human eye after 12 years. *Arch Ophthalmol* 1983;101:1399–1401.
43. Miyamoto K, Refojo MF, Tolentino FI, et al: Fluorinated oils as experimental vitreous substitutes. *Arch Ophthalmol* 1986;104:1053–1056.
44. Okun E: Intravitreal surgery utilizing liquid silicone: A long term followup. *Trans Pac Coast Oto-ophthalmol Soc* 1968;49:141–159.
45. Blodi FC: Injection and impregnation of liquid silicone into ocular tissues. *Am J Ophthalmol* 1971;71:1044–1051.
46. Laroche L, Pavlakis C, Saraux H, et al: Ocular findings following intravitreal silicone injection. *Arch Ophthalmol* 1983;101:1422–1425.
47. Honda Y, Ueno S, Miura M, et al: Silicone oil particles trapped in the subretinal space: Complications after substitution of the vitreous. *Ophthalmologica* 1986; 192:1–5.
48. Manschot WA: Intravitreal silicone injection. *Adv Ophthalmol* 1978;36:197–207.
49. Kirchhof B, Tavakolian U, Paulmann H, et al: Histopathological findings in eyes after silicone oil injection. *Graefes Arch Clin Exp Ophthalmol* 1986;224:34–37.
50. Parmley VC, Barishak R, Howes EL Jr, et al: Foreign-body giant cell reactions to liquid silicone. *Am J Ophthalmol* 1986;101:680–683.
51. Shikishima H, Ohki K, Machi N, et al: Effects and distribution of intravitreally or subretinally injected silicone oil identified in rabbit retina using osmium tetroxide method. *Jpn J Ophthalmol* 1992;36:469–478.
52. Shields CL, Eagle RC Jr: Pseudo-Schnabel's cavernous degeneration of the optic nerve secondary to intraocular silicone oil. *Arch Ophthalmol* 1989;107:714–717.
53. Suzuki M, Okada T, Takeuchi S, et al: Effect of silicone oil on ocular tissues. *Jpn J Ophthalmol* 1990;35:282–291.
54. Pastor JC, Lopez MI, Saornil MA, et al: Intravitreal silicone and fluorosilicone oils: Pathologic findings in rabbit eyes. *Acta Ophthalmol* 1992;70:651–658.
55. Meredith TA, Lindsey DT, Edelhauser HF, et al: Electroretinographic studies following vitrectomy and intraocular silicone oil injection. *Br J Ophthalmol* 1985; 69:254–260.
56. Thaler A, Lessel MR, Gnad H, et al: The influence of intravitreal injected silicone oil on electrophysiological potential of the eye. *Doc Ophthalmol* 1986;62:41–46.
57. Foerster MH, Esser J, Laqua H: Silicone oil and its influence on electrophysiologic findings. *Am J Ophthalmol* 1985;99:201–206.
58. Momirov D, Lith GHM van, Živojnović R: Electroretinogram and electrooculogram of eyes with intravitreously injected silicone oil. *Ophthalmologica* 1983; 186:183–188.
59. Refojo MF, Leong FL, Chung H, et al: Extraction of retinol and cholesterol by intraocular silicone oils. *Ophthalmology* 1988;95:614–618.

60. Leaver PK, Grey RHB, Garner A: Silicone oil injection in the treatment of massive preretinal retraction: II. Late complications in 93 eyes. *Br J Ophthalmol* 1979; 63:361–367.

61. Nakamura K, Refojo MF, Crabtree DV: Factors contributing to the emulsification of intraocular silicone and fluorosilicone oils. *Invest Ophthalmol Vis Sci* 1990;31:647–656.

62. Matsuda T: Surface chemistry of silicone oil as intraocular tamponade. *Acta Soc Ophthalmol Jpn* 1986;90:78.

63. Heidenkummer H-P, Kampik A, Thierfelder S: Experimentelle Untersuchungen zum sogenannten Emulsifikationsverhalten von Silikonöl: Einfluß der Viskosität. *Fortschr Ophthalmol* 1990;87:226–228.

64. Heidenkummer H-P, Kampik A, Thierfelder S: Emulsification of silicone oils with specific physicochemical characteristics. *Graefes Arch Clin Exp Ophthalmol* 1991;229:88–94.

65. Heidenkummer H-P, Kampik A, Thierfelder S: Experimental evaluation of in vitro stability of purified polydimethylsiloxanes (silicone oil) in viscosity ranges from 1000 to 5000 centistokes. *Retina* 1992;12(3 suppl):S28–S32.

66. Bartov E, Pennarola F, Savion N, et al: A quantitative in vitro model for silicone oil emulsification: Role of blood constituents. *Retina* 1992;12(3 suppl):S23–S27.

67. Lewis H, Burke JM, Abrams GW, et al: Perisilicone proliferation after vitrectomy for proliferative vitreoretinopathy. *Ophthalmology* 1988;94:583–591.

68. Charles S: *Vitreous Microsurgery*, 2nd ed. Baltimore: Williams & Wilkins, 1987, pp 146–147.

69. Lambrou FH, Burke JM, Aaberg TM: Effect of silicone oil on experimental traction retinal detachment. *Arch Ophthalmol* 1987;105:1269–1272.

70. Bottoni M, Sborgia M, Vinciguerra P, et al: Perfluorodecalin (PFD) and perfluorophenanthrene (PFP) as post-operative short-term vitreous substitutes. *J Vitreo Retina* 1992;1:37–41.

71. Lucke K, Laqua H: *Silicone Oil in the Treatment of Complicated Retinal Detachments: Techniques, Results and Complications*. New York: Springer-Verlag, 1990, pp 21–24.

72. Moisseiev J, Bartov E, Cahane M, et al: Cataract extraction in eyes filled with silicone oil. *Arch Ophthalmol* 1992;110:1649–1651.

73. Casswell AG, Gregor ZJ: Silicone oil removal: I. The effect on the complications of silicone oil. *Br J Ophthalmol* 1987;71:893–897.

74. Sternberg P Jr, Hatchell DL, Foulks GN, et al: The effect of silicone oil on the cornea. *Arch Ophthalmol* 1985;103:90–94.

75. Beekhuis WH, van Rij G, Živojnović R: Silicone oil keratopathy: Indications for keratoplasty. *Br J Ophthalmol* 1985;69:247–253.

76. McCuen BW II, De Juan E Jr, Landers MB III, et al: Silicone oil in vitreoretinal surgery: II. Results and complications. *Retina* 1985;5:198–205.

77. Setälä K, Ruusuvaara P, Punnonen E, et al: Changes in corneal endothelium after treatment of retinal detachment with intraocular silicone oil. *Acta Ophthalmol* 1989;67:37–43.

78. Lemmen KD, Michel K, Kirchhof B, et al: Klinische und Morphologische Aspekte der Silikon-Keratopathie im Tier-experiment. *Fortschr Ophthalmol* 1985;82: 556–558.

79. Gao R, Neubauer L, Tang S, et al: Silicone oil in the anterior chamber. *Graefes Arch Clin Exp Ophthalmol* 1989;227:106–109.

80. Karel I, Filipec M, Vrabec F, et al: The effect of liquid silicone on the corneal endothelium in rabbits. *Graefes Arch Clin Exp Ophthalmol* 1986;224:481–485.
81. Cairns JD, Anand N: Combined vitrectomy, intraocular microsurgery and liquid silicone in the treatment of proliferative vitreoretinopathy. *Aust J Ophthalmol* 1984;12:133–138.
82. Madreperla SA, McCuen BW: Rate of closure of surgical inferior peripheral iridectomy and effect of silicone oil position in eyes treated with silicone oil extended tamponade. *Invest Ophthalmol Vis Sci* 1994;35(Suppl):2071.
83. Zumbro DS, Waterhouse WJ, Wagner DG: The effects of silicone oil on in vitro laser iridotomy. *Invest Ophthalmol Vis Sci* 1994;35(Suppl):1616.
84. Haut J, Le Mer Y, Benrayana N, et al: Rétinotomies au laser YAG nano-seconde: A propos de 21 cas. *Bull Soc Ophtalmol Fr* 1988;88:1289–1291.
85. Huy CP, Larricart P, Warnet JM, et al: In vitro laser decomposition of silicone fluid used in detachment of the retina. *Ophthalmologica* 1992;204:23–26.
86. Leaver PK, Grey RH, Garner A: Complications following silicone-oil injection. *Mod Probl Ophthalmol* 1979;20:290–294.
87. Alexandridis E, Daniel H: Results of silicone oil injection into the vitreous. *Dev Ophthalmol* 1981;2:24–27.
88. Ando F: Intraocular hypertension resulting from pupillary block by silicone oil. *Am J Ophthalmol* 1985;99:87–88.
89. Živojnović R: *Silicone Oil in Vitreoretinal Surgery*. Dordrecht, The Netherlands: Martinus Nijhoff/Dr W Junk Pub, 1987, pp 130–133.
90. Laganowski HC, Leaver PK: Silicone oil in the aphakic eye: The influence of a six o'clock peripheral iridectomy. *Eye* 1989;3:338–348.
91. Zborowski-Gutman L, Treister G, Naveh N, et al: Acute glaucoma following vitrectomy and silicone oil injection. *Br J Ophthalmol* 1987;71:903–906.
92. Moisseiev J, Barak A, Manaim T, et al: Removal of silicone oil in the management of glaucoma in eyes with emulsified silicone. *Retina* 1993;13:290–295.
93. Weinberg RS, Peyman GA, Huamonte FU: Elevation of intraocular pressure after pars plana vitrectomy. *Albrecht von Graefes Arch Klin Ophthalmol* 1976; 200:157–161.
94. De Corral LR, Cohen SB, Peyman GA: Effect of intravitreal silicone oil on intraocular pressure. *Ophthalmic Surg* 1987;18:446–449.
95. Nguyen QH, Lloyd MA, Heuer DK, et al: Incidence and management of glaucoma after intravitreal silicone oil injection for complicated retinal detachments. *Ophthalmology* 1992;99:1520–1526.
96. Barr CC, Lai MY, Lean JS, et al: Postoperative intraocular pressure abnormalities in the Silicone Study. Silicone Study Report 4. *Ophthalmology* 1993; 100:1629–1635.
97. Silicone Study Group: Vitrectomy with silicone oil or sulfur hexafluoride gas in eyes with severe proliferative vitreoretinopathy: Results of a randomized clinical trial. *Arch Ophthalmol* 1992;110:770–779.
98. Casswell AG, Gregor ZJ: Silicone oil removal: II. Operative and postoperative complications. *Br J Ophthalmol* 1987;71:898–902.
99. Živojnović R, Mertens DAE, Peperkamp E: Das Flüssige Silikon in der Amotio chirurgie (II) Bericht über 280 Fälle-weitere Entwicklung der Technik. *Klin Monatsbl Augenheilkd* 1982;181:444–452.
100. Van Meurs JC, Mertens DAE, Peperkamp E, et al: Five-year results of vitrectomy

and silicone oil in patients with proliferative vitreoretinopathy. *Retina* 1993;
13:285–289.

101. Zilis JD, McCuen BW II, de Juan E Jr, et al: Results of silicone oil removal in
advanced proliferative vitreoretinopathy. *Am J Ophthalmol* 1989;108:15–21.

102. Cox MS, Trese MT, Murphy PL: Silicone oil for advanced proliferative vitreoretinopathy. *Ophthalmology* 1986;93:646–650.

103. Ando F, Miyake Y, Oshima K, et al: Temporary use of intraocular silicone oil in the
treatment of complicated retinal detachment. *Graefes Arch Clin Exp Ophthalmol*
1986;224:32–33.

104. Kampik A, Hoing C, Heidenkummer HP: Problems and timing in the removal of
silicone oil. *Retina* 1992;12:S11–S16.

105. Haller JA, Campochiaro PA: Oil and gas on troubled waters: The proliferative vitreoretinopathy studies. *Arch Ophthalmol* 1992;110:769–770.

106. Silicone Study Group: Vitrectomy with silicone oil or perfluoropropane gas in eyes
with severe proliferative vitreoretinopathy: Results of a randomized clinical study:
Silicone Study Report 2. *Arch Ophthalmol* 1992;110:780–792.

107. Hutchinson AK, Capone A, Grossenklaus HE: Subconjunctival silicone oil after
vitreoretinal surgery. *Am J Ophthalmol* 1993;115:109–110.

108. Gonvers M: Temporary silicone oil tamponade in the management of retinal
detachment with proliferative vitreoretinopathy. *Am J Ophthalmol* 1985;100:
239–245.

109. Johnson RN, Flynn HW Jr, Parel J-M, et al: Transient hypopyon with marked anterior chamber fibrin following pars plana vitrectomy and silicone oil injection.
Arch Ophthalmol 1989;107:683–686.

110. De Corral LR, Peyman GA: Silicone oil injection in aphakic eyes: A modified technique. *Ophthalmic Surg* 1985;16:774–775.

111. Gnad H, Skorpik C, Paroussis P, et al: Funktionelle und anatomische Resultate
nach temporärey Silikon ölimplantation. *Klin Monatsbl Augenheilkd* 1984;
185:364–367.

112. Ruellan Y-M, Roussat B: Décollement de rétine: Tamponnement interne provisoire
par huile de silicone après vitrectomie: Résultats anatomiques et fonctionnels. *J Fr
Ophtalmol* 1985;8:117–124.

113. Gonvers M: Temporary use of intraocular silicone oil in the treatment of detachment with massive periretinal proliferation: Preliminary report. *Ophthalmologica*
1982;184:210–218.

114. Kampik A, Gabel VP, Spiegel D: Intraokulare Tamponade mit hochviskösem
Silikonöl bei massiver proliferativer Vitreo-Retinopathie. *Klin Monatsbl Augenheilkd* 1984;185:368–370.

115. Barthelemy F, Chauvaud D, Frota A: Utilisation de l'huile de silicone en tamponnement transitoire dans le traitement des décollements de rétine avec rétraction
vitréo-rétinienne: I. Résultats anatomiques et fonctionnels à court et long termes
sur 110 cas. *J Fr Ophtalmol* 1984;7:273–277.

116. Laqua H, Lucke K, Foerster MH: Entwicklung und gegenwärtiger Stand der
Silikonölchirurgie. *Klin Monatsbl Augenheilkd* 1988;192:277–283.

117. Haut J, Ullern M, Chatellier P, et al: Resultats de 200 cas d'injection intraoculaire
de silicone associee a la vitrectomie. *Bull Mem Soc Fr Ophtalmol* 1979;
91:180–184.

118. Heimann K, Dimopoulos S, Paulmann H: Silikonolinjektion in der Behandlung
komplizierter Netzhautablösungen. *Klin Monatsbl Augenheilkd* 1984;185:
505–508.

119. Haut J, Van Effenterre G, Flamand M: Treatment of macular hole retinal detachment with silicone oil, with or without argon laser photocoagulation. *Ophthalmologica* 1983;187:25–28.

120. Bacin F, Gibert C: Résultats du traitement des décollements de rétine avec rétraction du vitré par injections de silicone liquide intra-oculaire. *Bull Soc Ophthalmol Fr* 1982;82:367–372.

121. McCuen BW II, De Juan E, Machemer R: Silicone oil in vitreoretinal surgery: I. Surgical techniques. *Retina* 1989;5:189–197.

122. Živojnović R: *Silicone Oil in Vitreoretinal Surgery.* Dordrecht, The Netherlands: Martinus Nijhoff/Dr W Junk Pub, 1987, pp 25–28.

123. Maberly AL, Antworth MV: The use of silicone oil in vitreoretinal surgery. *Can J Ophthalmol* 1989;24:265–268.

124. Grisolano J, Peyman GA: Special short needles to inject and aspirate high-viscosity silicone oil. *Arch Ophthalmol* 1986;104:608.

125. Peyman GA, De Corral LR: One-step extracapsular cataract extraction and silicone oil-injection in the management of proliferative vitreoretinopathy. *Br J Ophthalmol* 1986;70:382–386.

126. Bartov E, Ginsburg LH, Hirsh A, et al: Methylcellulose as a contact lens irrigant when silicone oil is used in vitreoretinal surgery. *Ann Ophthalmol* 1993; 25:167–169.

127. Yeo JH, Glaser BM, Michels RG: Silicone oil in the treatment of complicated retinal detachments. *Ophthalmology* 1987;94:1109–1113.

128. Živojnović R: *Silicone Oil in Vitreoretinal Surgery.* Dordrecht, The Netherlands: Martinus Nijhoff/Dr W Junk Pub, 1987, p 269.

129. Unosson K, Stenkula S, Törnqvist P, et al: Liquid silicone in the treatment of retinal detachment. *Acta Ophthalmol* 1985;63:656–660.

130. Leaver PK, Lean JS: Management of giant retinal tears using vitrectomy and silicone oil/fluid exchange: A preliminary report. *Trans Ophthalmol Soc UK* 1981; 101:189–191.

131. Fletcher ME, Peyman GA: A simplified technique for the removal of liquid silicone from vitrectomized eyes. *Retina* 1987;5:168–171.

132. Živojnović R: *Silicone Oil in Vitreoretinal Surgery.* Dordrecht, The Netherlands: Martinus Nijhoff/Dr W Junk Pub, 1987, pp 60–69.

133. Lean JS: Use of silicone oil as an additional technique in vitreoretinal surgery, in Ryan SJ (ed): *Retina,* vol 3, *Surgical Retina.* St. Louis: CV Mosby, 1989, pp 279–292.

134. Leaver PK, Cooling RJ, Feretis EB, et al: Vitrectomy and fluid/silicone-oil exchange for giant retinal tears: Results at six months. *Br J Ophthalmol* 1984;68:432–438.

135. Murray TG, Boldt HC, Lewis H, et al: A technique for facilitated visualization and dissection of the vitreous base, pars plana, and pars plicata. *Arch Ophthalmol* 1991;109:1458–1459.

136. Billington BM, Leaver PK: Vitrectomy and fluid/silicone-oil exchange for giant retinal tears: Results at 18 months. *Graefes Arch Clin Exp Ophthalmol* 1986; 224:7–10.

137. Michels RG, Wilkinson SP, Rice TA: *Retinal Detachment.* St. Louis: CV Mosby, 1990, pp 625–760.

138. Ando F, Kondo J: Surgical techniques for giant retinal tears with retinal tacks. *Ophthalmic Surg* 1986;17:408–411.

139. Stilma JS, Koster R, Živojnović R: Radical vitrectomy and silicone-oil injection in

the treatment of proliferative vitreoretinopathy following retinal detachment. *Doc Ophthalmol* 1986;64:109–116.

140. Stern WH, Johnson RN, Irvine AR, et al: Extended retinal tamponade in the treatment of retinal detachment with proliferative vitreoretinopathy. *Br J Ophthalmol* 1986;70:911–917.

141. Kroll P, Berg P, Biermeyer H: Langzeitergebnisse nach vitreoretinaler Silikonölchirurgie. *Fortschr Ophthalmol* 1988;85:259–262.

142. Lucke KH, Föerster MH, Laqua H: Long-term results of vitrectomy and silicone oil in 500 cases of complicated retinal detachments. *Am J Ophthalmol* 1987;104:624–633.

143. Yeo JH, Glaser BM, Michels RG: Silicone oil in the treatment of complicated retinal detachments. *Ophthalmology* 1987;94:1109–1113.

144. Sell CH, McCuen BW II, Landers MB III, et al: Long-term results of successful vitrectomy with silicone oil for advanced proliferative vitreoretinopathy. *Am J Ophthalmol* 1987;103:24–28.

145. Roussat B, Ruellan YM: Traitement du décollement de rétine par vitrectomie et injection d'huile de silicone: Résultats à long terme et complications dans 105 cas. *J Fr Ophtalmol* 1984;7:11–18.

146. Fisher YL, Shakin JL, Slakter JS, et al: Perfluoropropane gas, modified panretinal photocoagulation and vitrectomy in the management of severe proliferative vitreoretinopathy. *Arch Ophthalmol* 1988;106:1255–1260.

147. Fisher YL, Shakin JL, Slakter JS, et al: Peripheral panretinal photocoagulation and perfluoropropane/air mixture in vitreoretinal surgery for proliferative vitreoretinopathy. *Dev Ophthalmol* 1985;11:194–199.

148. Bonnet M, Santamaria E, Mouche J: Intraoperative use of pure perfluoropropane gas in the management of proliferative vitreoretinopathy. *Graefes Arch Clin Exp Ophthalmol* 1987;225:299–302.

149. Chang S, Lincoff HA, Coleman DJ, et al: Perfluorocarbon gases in vitreous surgery. *Ophthalmology* 1985;92:651–656.

150. Stirpe M, Orciuolo M: Vitrectomy, scleral buckling, and peripheral diathermy treatment for severe proliferative vitreoretinopathy. *Retina* 1987;7:219–222.

151. Riedel KG, Gabel V-P, Neubauer L, et al: Intravitreal silicone oil injection: Complications and treatment of 415 consecutive patients. *Graefes Arch Clin Exp Ophthalmol* 1990;228:19–23.

152. Aaberg TM: Management of anterior and posterior proliferative vitreoretinopathy. *Am J Ophthalmol* 1988;106:519–532.

153. Peyman GA, Kao GW, de Corral LR: Randomized clinical trial of intraocular silicone vs gas in the management of complicated retinal detachment and vitreous hemorrhage. *Int Ophthalmol* 1987;10:221–234.

154. Stern WH, Fisher SK, Anderson DH, et al: Epiretinal membrane formation after vitrectomy. *Am J Ophthalmol* 1982;93:757–772.

155. Scott JD: The treatment of massive vitreous retraction. *Trans Ophthalmol Soc UK* 1973;93:417–423.

156. Grey RHB, Leaver PK: Silicone oil in the treatment of massive pre-retinal proliferation: I. Results in 105 eyes. *Br J Ophthalmol* 1979;63:355–360.

157. Diddie KR, Stern WH, Ober RR, et al: Intraocular silicone oil for recurrent proliferative vitreoretinopathy in vitrectomized eyes. *Invest Ophthalmol Vis Sci* 1983;24(suppl):173.

158. Skorpik C, Menapace R, Gnad HD, et al: Silicone oil implantation in penetrating injuries complicated by PVR: Results from 1982 to 1986. *Retina* 1989;9:8–14.

159. McLeod D: Silicone-oil injection during closed microsurgery for diabetic retinal detachment. *Graefes Arch Clin Exp Ophthalmol* 1986;224:55–59.

160. Sternberg P Jr, Meredith T: Management of recurrent retinal detachment after silicone oil injection. *Arch Ophthalmol* 1987;105:27–28.

161. Lucke K, Föerster M, Laqua H: Langzeiterfahrungen mit intraokularer Silikonöl-Füllung. *Fortschr Ophthalmol* 1987;84:96–98.

162. Kirkby GR, Gregor ZJ: The removal of silicone oil from the anterior chamber in phakic eyes. *Arch Ophthalmol* 1987;105:1592.

163. Beekhuis WH, Ando F, Živojnović R, et al: Basal iridectomy at 6 o'clock in the aphakic eye treated with silicone oil: Prevention of keratopathy and secondary glaucoma. *Br J Ophthalmol* 1987;71:197–200.

164. Elliott AJ, Bacon AS, Scott JD: The superior peripheral iridectomy: Prevention of pupil block due to silicone oil. *Eye* 1990;4:226–229.

165. McCuen BW II, Zen SP, Stern W, et al: Vitrectomy with silicone oil or perfluoropropane gas in eyes with severe proliferative vitreoretinopathy: Silicone Study Report No. 3. *Retina* 1993;13:279–284.

166. Blumenkranz MS, Azen SP, Aaberg T, et al: Relaxing retinotomy with silicone oil or long acting gas in eyes with severe proliferative vitreoretinopathy: Silicone Study Report 5. *Am J Ophthalmol* 1993;116:557–564.

167. Araiz JJ, Refojo MF, Arroyo MH, et al: Antiproliferative effect of retinoic acid in intravitreous silicone oil in an animal model of proliferative vitreoretinopathy. *Invest Ophthalmol Vis Sci* 1993;34:522–530.

168. Manzanas L, Marin J, Refojo MF: Retinol in silicone oil for treating proliferative vitreoretinopathy. *Invest Ophthalmol Vis Sci* 1990;31(Suppl):24.

169. Arroyo MH, Refojo MF, Araiz JJ, et al: Silicone oil as a delivery vehicle for BCNU in rabbit proliferative vitreoretinopathy. *Retina* 1993;13:245–250.

170. Heimenn K, Dahl B, Dimopoulos S, et al: Pars plana vitrectomy and silicone oil injection in proliferative diabetic retinopathy. *Graefes Arch Clin Exp Ophthalmol* 1989;227:152–156.

171. Rinkoff JS, de Juan E Jr, McCuen BW II: Silicone oil for retinal detachment with advanced proliferative vitreoretinopathy following failed vitrectomy for proliferative diabetic retinopathy. *Am J Ophthalmol* 1986;101:181–186.

172. De Corral LR, Peyman GA: Pars plana vitrectomy and intravitreal silicone oil injection in eyes with rubeosis irides. *Can J Ophthalmol* 1986;21:10–12.

173. Ohrt V: The frequency of rubeosis iridis in diabetic patients. *Acta Ophthalmol* 1971;49:301–307.

174. Blankenship G: Preoperative iris rubeosis and diabetic vitrectomy results. *Ophthalmology* 1980;87:176–182.

175. Blankenship GW: The lens influence on diabetic vitrectomy results: Report of a prospective randomized study. *Arch Ophthalmol* 1980;98:2196–2198.

176. Aiello LM, Wand M, Liang G: Anterior and posterior segment neovascularization following cataract extraction in patients with diabetes mellitus. *Ophthalmology* 1982;89(suppl):115.

177. Rice TA, Michels RG, Maguire MG, et al: The effect of lensectomy on the incidence of iris neovascularization and neovascular glaucoma after vitrectomy for diabetic retinopathy. *Am J Ophthalmol* 1986;95:1–11.

178. Schachat AP, Oyakawa RT, Michels RG, et al: Complications of vitreous surgery for diabetic retinopathy. *Ophthalmology* 1983;90(5):522–529.

179. Brourman ND, Blumenkranz MS, Cox MS, et al: Silicone oil for the treatment of severe proliferative diabetic retinopathy. *Ophthalmology* 1989;96:759–764.

180. Glaser BM, D'Amore PA, Michels RG, et al: Demonstration of vasoproliferative activity from mammalian retina. *J Cell Biol* 1980;84:298–304.
181. Azzolini C, Brancato R, Camesasca FI, et al: Influence of silicone oil on iris microangiopathy in diabetic vitrectomized eyes. *Ophthalmology* 1993;100: 1152–1159.
182. McCuen BW II, Rinkoff JS: Silicone oil for progressive anterior ocular neovascularization after failed diabetic vitrectomy. *Arch Ophthalmol* 1989;107:677–682.
183. Barry PJ, Hiscott PS, Grierson I, et al: Reparative epiretinal fibrosis after diabetic vitrectomy. *Trans Ophthalmol Soc UK* 1985;104:283–296.
184. Wilson-Holt N, Gregor Z: Spontaneous relieving retinotomies in diabetic silicone filled eyes. *Eye* 1992;6:461–464.
185. Zaubosma H, Hemo I: Silicone oil tamponade for retinal detachment and delayed treatment of retinal tears. *Ophthalmic Surg* 1993;24:600–693.
186. Blankenship GW: Management of vitreous cavity hemorrhage following pars plana vitrectomy for diabetic retinopathy. *Ophthalmology* 1986;93:39–44.
187. Pearson RV, Hebard D, Gregor ZJ: Removal of silicone following diabetic vitrectomy. *Br J Ophthalmol* 1993;77:204–207.

Chapter 2
Intraocular Gases

Intraocular gas has many uses in vitreous and retinal detachment surgery. Gas can tamponade retinal tears until a permanent chorioretinal adhesion forms to seal them. Such tamponading of a retinal tear increases reabsorption of subretinal fluid and decreases the amount of indentation necessary in the placement of encircling bands and radial sponges. Postoperative hypotony with the sequela of choroidal effusion can be prevented by restoring intraocular volume. Restoring the intraocular volume reduces the amount of induced astigmatism, myopia, and ocular deformity. Retinal folds, including fishmouthing of horseshoe tears placed on a buckle, may be eliminated by the internal splinting effect of intraocular gas.

The use of intraocular gas, however, may cause various complications. Intraocular injection can introduce impurities or pathogens into the eye. The lens or retina may be penetrated by the needle used for injection, and expansion of gases may raise intraocular pressure (IOP) and occlude the central retinal artery. If postoperative positioning is improper, pupillary block glaucoma may result. Moreover, contact of the gas with the lens may initiate cataract formation, and inadvertent injection of many small gas bubbles may impede examination of the fundus.

AIR

Air, the first gas injected intraocularly, was used by Ohm in 1911.[1] He was unaware of the tamponading effect on the retinal tear and used intraocular air only to hold the retina in position. Ohm described four cases of retinal detachment that he treated by puncturing the sclera, draining the subretinal fluid, and injecting air into the vitreous cavity to force the retina back into position against the choroid. Two of his four cases were successful.

In 1938, Rosengren[2] reported the first of a series of six cases of rhegmatogenous retinal detachment that he treated similarly. He injected air into the vitreous body after diathermy had been performed around the retinal hole. After the operation, the patient was carefully positioned so that the tear was situated superiorly. The rising air bubble pressed the retina against the choroid in the diathermized area. In subsequent publications,[3,4] Rosengren described a total of 256 cases treated in this manner. He reported that nearly all of the injected air (1.5 to 2.0 mL) was reabsorbed within 8 days. Of these 256 cases, 198 retinas were reattached using this procedure.

Other investigators[5,6] have supported the use of intravitreal air for superior detachments. Arruga[7] subsequently proposed the use of this technique to treat a variety of retinal detachments. Pillat,[8] however, believed that the use of air injection is more beneficial for the treatment of inferiorly located detachments, whereby the rising air bubble forces the formed vitreous down to tamponade the inferior detachment.

In 1969, Norton and co-workers[9] reported clinical success, and Machemer and associates[10] described experimental success using intravitreal air injection to manage giant retinal tears. However, the air remains in the eye for only a short period and does not expand after intraocular injection.

In 1959, Schenk[11] evaluated the use in intraocular injection of oxygen, nitrogen, carbon dioxide, and argon. He found that nitrogen remained in the vitreous of rabbits for the longest time before being resorbed (60 hours for 2 mL and 42 hours for 1 mL) and correlated this finding with the solubility of these gases in water. A similar study by Widder in 1962,[12] evaluating argon, krypton, and radon, showed that argon was the most slowly absorbed gas, as suggested by the lower solubility of argon in water. However, other studies have demonstrated that all the inert gases are absorbed more rapidly than air, thus offering no advantage.[13,14]

PRINCIPLES INVOLVED IN EXPANSION AND ABSORPTION OF LONG-ACTING GASES

The expansion and longevity of various intravitreal gas bubbles increases with the insolubility of the selected gas in aqueous fluid.[15] Gases present in the tissue (mainly nitrogen) enter the gas bubble faster than the long-acting gas is reabsorbed. This is the primary reason intravitreal gas bubbles initially expand.

According to one theory,[16-18] three stages of gas dynamics are differentiated after injection of a pure long-acting gas bubble into the eye (Fig. 2–1A,B).[19,20] These stages are affected by both diffusion and convection.[15] The initial phase[19,20] starts when the pure gas is injected intravitreally and continues until the pure gas diffuses out of the bubble because of a pressure gradient. Diffusion is slow because of a low diffusion coefficient, low water solubility, and high molecular weight.[20,21] In contrast, because of a partial pressure gradient, oxygen, carbon dioxide, and nitrogen diffuse rapidly into the gas bubble from the surrounding fluid, and an equilibration of the first two gases is quickly achieved.[18,19] A rapid influx of nitrogen into the bubble, which is much greater than the efflux of the long-acting gas from the bubble, causes an early expansion of the gas bubble[15,22] and a decrease in the concentration of the long-acting gas in the intravitreal gas pocket.

Figure 2–1. A. Variation in concentration in a rabbit intravitreal gas pocket with time. Initial volume and concentration injected were 0.85 cc 100% SF_6. **B.** Theoretical summary of the gas dynamics of an intravitreal gas SF_6 pocket. Theoretical values—Tenny, Carpenter, & Rahn. J. Applied Physiol 6:201, 1953. ( ) Experimental values, † Atmospheric pressure plus 10P 15 nm Hg, ‡ Volume as measured at atmospheric pressure , ≢ Average right heart measurements plus 10P 15 nm Hg (From Abrams GW, Edelhauser HF, Aaberg TM, et al: Dynamics of intravitreal SF_6 gas. *Invest Ophthalmol* 1974;13:863–868.)

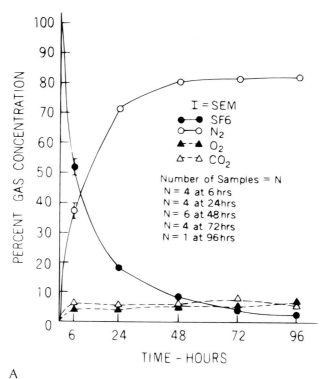

A

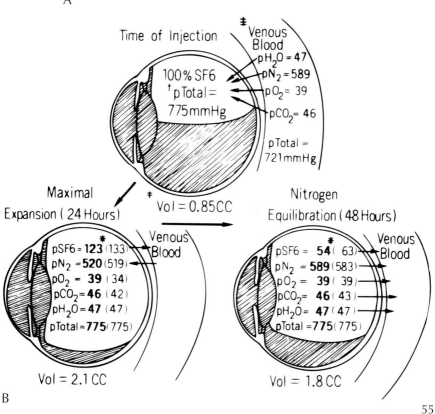

B

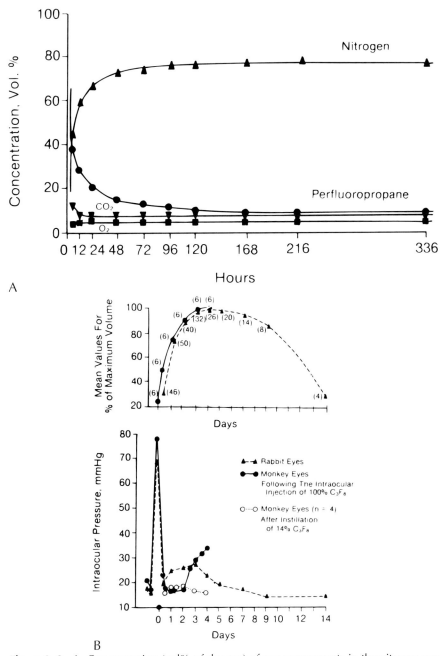

A

B

Figure 2–2. A. Concentration (vol% of dry gas) of gas components in the vitreous cavity after instillation of 0.4 mL perfluoropropane at zero time. **B.** Mean percent of maximum bubble volume (above) and mean IOP (below) after instillation of perfluoropropane into rabbit and monkey eyes. (From Peters MA, Abrams GW, Hamilton LH, et al: The nonexpansile, equilibrated concentration of perfluoropropane gas in the eye. *Am J Ophthalmol* 1985;100:831–839. Published with permission from the American Journal of Ophthalmology. Copyright by the Ophthalmic Publishing Company.)

The second phase starts at the point of maximal expansion and continues until the nitrogen partial pressures in the gas bubble and capillary blood reach equilibrium.[19,20] This transitional stage[19] is marked by a decrease in the partial pressure gradient for nitrogen, because nitrogen has already entered the bubble, and long-acting gas has left it (Fig. 2–2). As a result, expansion of the intravitreal gas bubble not only stops, but a slow reabsorption begins.[20] Because of a large pressure gradient, the long-acting gas leaves the intraocular bubble at a faster rate than nitrogen enters, despite the lower water solubility and diffusion rate of the gas.[15,20]

The last phase is initiated when nitrogen pressure in the gas bubble exceeds or equilibrates with the capillary nitrogen pressure.[19,20] This third phase is marked by a diffusion of all gases from the bubble and a gradual reduction in the gas bubble volume. A stable concentration of all gases in the intraocular bubble is achieved, which is maintained during the subsequent efflux of gases from the bubble.

Crittenden et al[15] demonstrated in animal experiments that convection currents involving the surrounding fluid, rather than diffusion, are the main determinant of the early expansion of a long-acting gas bubble. The type of long-acting gas is not a significant factor in the early phase of expansion, which may explain why the intravitreal expansion rates of sulfur hexafluoride (SF_6) and perfluoropropane (C_3F_8) are similar despite differences in the rates of nitrogen diffusion into these two gases.[20] Animal experiments[23] have also demonstrated that SF_6 and octafluorocyclobutane expand at nearly the same rate during the early phase of expansion.

Different factors affect convection, including aphakia, vitrectomy, and eye movement.[15] Crittenden demonstrated experimentally that diffusion differs in eyes that have and have not undergone vitrectomy.[15] These differences account for a variability in gas expansion and disappearance in eyes filled with similar volumes of intravitreal gas.

To use an intraocular gas bubble of sufficient duration and size to tamponade a retinal tear, the kinetics of different gases must be understood and the location of the retinal breaks considered. A small to medium-sized bubble can more easily tamponade a superior or posterior break than an inferior one.

LONG-ACTING GASES

Sulfur Hexafluoride (SF_6)

Investigators sought a gas that would expand in the eye when only small volumes could be injected and would remain in the eye longer than air and work as an internal tamponade to push the retina against the retinal pigment epithelium (RPE) until chorioretinal scarring occurred. Two gases met these criteria: SF_6 and octafluorocyclobutane (C_4F_8).[13] Lincoff and associates[24] and Norton[25] described the properties of SF_6 for intraocular injection (Fig. 2–3). A colorless gas of high molecular weight, SF_6 has poor solubility in water, is inert, and has a poor diffusion coefficient. These characteristics enable it to be retained in the eye for a considerably longer period than air. Because the gas diffuses poorly out of the eye, nitrogen, oxygen, and car-

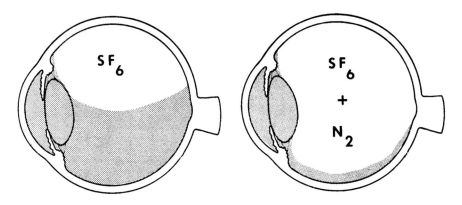

Figure 2–3. Expansion of gas bubble immediately after injection (left) and 48 hours later (right). (From Norton EWD: Intraocular gas in the management of selected retinal detachments. *Trans Am Acad Ophthalmol Otolaryngol* 1973;77:OP85-OP98.)

bon dioxide are diffused into the eye to reach an equilibrium that expands the initial volume of SF_6 used. Norton[25] demonstrated that 2 mL was the maximum amount of pure SF_6 that could be injected intraocularly without causing a significant pressure elevation. Aaberg and colleagues[26] found that an intraocular injection containing more than 18% SF_6 expands. Despite expansion, these investigators noted that the vitreous cavity can be safely filled with up to a 40:60 mixture of SF_6 and air without affecting IOP.

In rabbit experiments, after removing approximately 40% of the vitreous, Killey and associates[23] found that replacement with an equal volume of 100% SF_6 or 100% C_4F_8 resulted in a pressure increase of more than 20 mm Hg and loss of the remaining vitreous volume. This pressure increase occurred within 2 hours of injection. A mixture of 40% SF_6 and 60% air had no effect on pressure. When 20% of the vitreous volume in rabbits was substituted with either 100% SF_6 or 100% C_4F_8, no increase in IOP was recorded, but loss of vitreous volume equaled 2 times the amount of SF_6 injected and 3 times the C_4F_8. Significant loss of vitreous volume was found in eyes with elevated IOP as well as in eyes with intravitreal gas pockets (40% SF_6) but no similar increase in IOP. These investigators found that loss of vitreous volume was linear, with volume decreasing as the gas bubble expanded. This was true of SF_6 and C_4F_8. At 24 hours, loss was measured at 0.96 ± 0.06 g for C_4F_8, 0.68 ± 0.07 g for 100% SF_6, and 0.46 ± 0.08 g for 40% SF_6.

Absorption of SF_6 takes almost twice as long as air[27] (10 to 11 days versus 5 to 6 days), which permits a stronger chorioretinal adhesion to form.

Cataracts and keratopathy have developed after intraocular injection of SF_6. Experiments on owl monkeys demonstrated that cataracts resulted only when SF_6 remained in contact with the lens,[27] a complication that can be avoided by proper positioning of the patient. The cataracts were considered to be caused by the mechanical effect of SF_6, and they could be reproduced by exposing the lens to air. Electroretinograms (ERGs) performed on monkey eyes injected with SF_6 and control eyes showed similar findings. Light and electron microscopy demonstrated no evidence of retinal damage when comparing normal SF_6-filled with air-filled eyes. Both the air-filled and SF_6-filled eyes demonstrated some thickening of the outer segments of the retina. However, this finding was considered to be nonspecific. Van Horn and associates[28] demonstrated corneal endothelial changes and duplication of Descemet's membrane in rabbit eyes exposed to either SF_6 or air (Figs. 2–4, 2–5). After intraocular resorption of SF_6 or air, corneal morphology returned to normal. The investigators indicated that SF_6 did not appear to have direct toxic effects on the cornea. Their findings suggested that any gas in contact with the endothelium would cause similar changes.[28]

Two reports[29,30] emphasized that caution must be exercised when using SF_6. Sabates and colleagues[29] reported a series of 69 retinal detachment cases without vitrectomy in which SF_6 was used. Twenty-seven percent of the patients developed a transient elevation of IOP on the first postoperative day. Four eyes had central retinal artery occlusions. Three of the patients were diabetic. Sabates et al attributed the arterial occlusions to the effects of vascular disease and increased IOP. Killey and

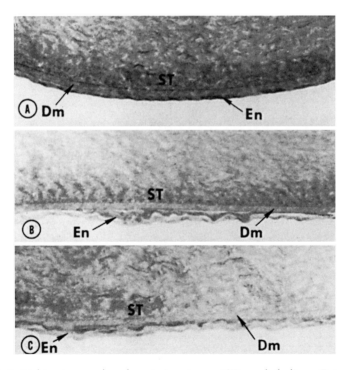

Figure 2–4. Light micrographs of posterior stroma (ST), endothelium (En), and Descemet's membrane (Dm) of: **A.** Control, sham-injected cornea; **B.** Cornea exposed to SF_6; and **C.** Cornea exposed to air for 3 days. The endothelium is multilayered in both of the experimental corneas. (All × 280). (From Van Horn DL, Edelhauser HF, Aaberg TM, et al: In vivo effects of air and sulfur hexafluoride gas on rabbit corneal endothelium. *Invest Ophthalmol* 1972;11:1028–1036.)

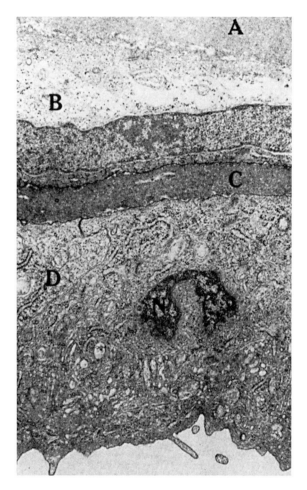

Figure 2–5. Endothelium 3 days after the injection of SF_6. The original Descemet's membrane **(A)** and endothelial cell layer **(B)** are covered by recently formed Descemet's membrane–like material **(C)** and a second endothelial cell layer **(D)**. Note the disorganized appearance of the original endothelial cell ($\times$ 10,500). (From Van Horn DL, Edelhauser HF, Aaberg TM, et al: In vivo effects of air and sulfur hexafluoride gas on rabbit corneal endothelium. *Invest Ophthalmol* 1972;11:1028–1036.)

associates[23] demonstrated an increase in IOP 6 hours after injection of SF_6 into animal eyes. They recommended measuring the pressure in all patients 4 to 6 hours after surgery. Abrams and colleagues[30] described 101 vitrectomies in 94 patients in whom intravitreal SF_6 was used. On the first postoperative day, 11 eyes had probable central retinal arterial occlusion with no light perception. Ten of these patients had intraocular complications, with nine experiencing severe vitreous hemorrhage. Abrams et al concluded that extensive vitreous hemorrhage should preclude the use of intraocular gas. If the outflow is compromised, eyes are more likely to develop increased IOP. A correlation was found between eyes that received 100% SF_6 and increased IOP, but no relationship was demonstrated between the volume of gas injected and IOP.

Perfluorocarbon Gases

Perfluorocarbon gases have been studied in both animals[13,23,31-35] and humans,[36,37] although their original use was as refrigerants and insulators. These gases are very insoluble, limiting their ability to cross the blood–aqueous barrier and leave the eye. This property results in sustained intraocular longevity compared with air, thus increasing the time they are able to tamponade retinal tears effectively.

Compared with SF_6, perfluorocarbon gases have an increased expansion and persistence, resulting in a smaller volume being required for intraocular injection. A small increase in IOP may occur after initial intravitreal injection of a perfluorocarbon. These gases have longer half-lives than SF_6, allowing a more prolonged internal tamponade.[35]

Octafluorocyclobutane (C_4F_8). An inert, high-molecular-weight gas that is poorly soluble in water, C_4F_8 has a low diffusion coefficient. Early work by Vygantas and co-workers[13] demonstrated that C_4F_8 expands more and remains inside the eye longer than does SF_6 (Table 2–1). Whereas 100% SF_6 expands to twice its volume, 100% C_4F_8 expands to 3 times the volume injected,[23] remains in the eye 50% longer than SF_6, and provides a longer tamponade of the retina against the RPE.[13] Rabbit experiments by Killey and associates[23] showed a significant increase of 20 mm Hg within 2 hours after injecting both 100% C_4F_8 and 100% SF_6 in rabbit eyes. From 18 to 24 hours after injection, the pressure elevation was significantly higher in eyes containing C_4F_8.

Vygantas and associates[13] histologically studied rabbit eyes after C_4F_8 injection, and no evidence of toxicity was found. Clinical and histologic studies of owl

TABLE 2–1. NUMBER OF EYES INJECTED WITH EACH GAS AND PERCENTAGE OF EYES CONTAINING GAS FOR EACH DAY AFTER INJECTION

Gas	No. of Eyes Injected	Eyes Containing Gas (%) *										
		1	2	3	4	5	6	7	8	9	10	11
Air	80	98	73	1								
Xenon	10	80	0									
Argon	10	90	10	0								
Krypton	10	90	20	0								
Helium	10	100	70	0								
Neon	10	100	90	0								
SF_6	14	100	100	86	71	21	0					
C_4F_8	16	100	100	100	100	94	75	63	50	44	13	0

*According to days postinjection. (From Vygantas CM, Peyman GA, Daily MJ, et al: Octafluorocyclobutane and other gases for vitreous replacement. *Arch Ophthalmol* 1973;90:235-236.)

monkey eyes after intravitreal C_4F_8 injection showed no evidence of toxicity except for the formation of posterior subcapsular cataracts in all eyes receiving more than 1.5 mL pure gas and one eye receiving a 1.5-mL mixture of 40% C_4F_8 and air (Fig. 2–6).[33] Eyes injected with smaller volumes of either pure C_4F_8 or a mixture of gases did not develop cataracts. The cataracts were probably caused by the mechanical irritation of the lens rather than direct toxicity of C_4F_8. Another study[32] compared the toxicity and duration of C_4F_8, air, and SF_6. Injections into the anterior chambers of rabbits showed that a volume of 0.15 mL caused increased IOP leading to buphthalmos and transitory corneal opacification (Fig. 2–7A, B). Smaller volumes or 40% mixtures of these gases with air caused minimal toxicity to the anterior chamber structure. Additionally, C_4F_8 consistently remained in the eye longer than SF_6 or air. Taylor and co-workers[31] demonstrated that breathing fluorinated hydrocarbon can cause cardiac arrhythmias. Tests on owl monkeys after C_4F_8 injection did not demonstrate any such irregularities.[33]

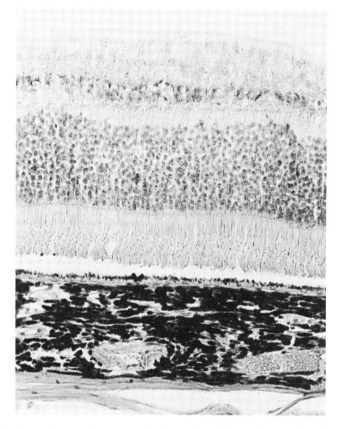

Figure 2–6. Normal retina 1 month after injection of 1.5 mL pure C_4F_8 (hematoxylin-eosin, × 250). (Peyman GA, Vygantas CM, Bennett TO, et al: Octafluorocyclobutane in vitreous and aqueous humor replacement. *Arch Ophthalmol* 1975;93:514–517. Copyright 1975, American Medical Association.)

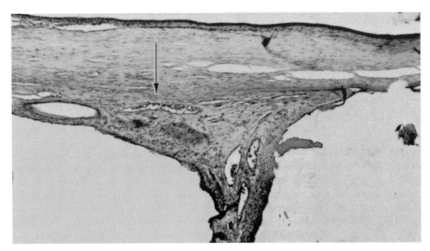

A

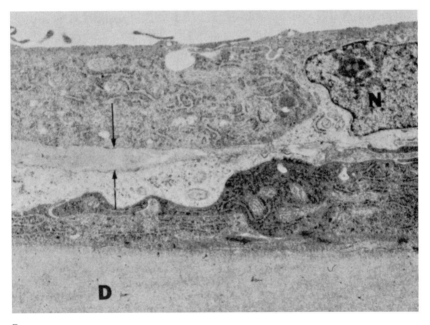

B

Figure 2–7. A. Magnified view of anterior chamber of eye 2 weeks after injection of 0.15 mL C_4F_8. Note peripheral anterior synechiae and end of Descemet's membrane (arrow) (hematoxylin-eosin, $\times$ 25). **B.** Two layers of endothelial cells with production of Descemet's membrane material (arrows). Specimen was taken from cornea over 0.15-cc pure C_4F_8 bubble and shows nucleus of endothelial cells (N) and Descemet membrane (D) (original magnification, $\times$ 12,500). (From Brubaker S, Peyman GA, Vygantas C: Toxicity of octafluorocyclobutane after intracameral injection. *Arch Ophthalmol* 1974;92:324–328. Copyright 1974; American Medical Association.)

Peyman and associates[37] injected a mixture of C_4F_8 and air in 12 patients undergoing repair of retinal detachment. Treatment consisted of intravitreal gas injection combined with intrascleral diathermy. The mixture of 40% C_4F_8 and 60% air injected intravitreally in volumes of 0.5 to 4.0 mL remained inside the eyes for periods ranging from 12 to 30 days. No postoperative complications were encountered, except for one case of glaucoma that required release of gas and a case of mild postoperative iritis when 4 mL gas mixture was used.

Working with albino rabbit eyes, Peyman and associates[33] studied the composition of pure C_4F_8 after intravitreal injection. Twenty-four and forty-eight hours after injection of 0.1 mL pure C_4F_8 in the vitreous, the presence of oxygen, nitrogen, and carbon dioxide was shown by gas chromatographic analysis (Table 2–2). This finding supports the hypothesis of volume expansion secondary to diffusion of above-mentioned gases inside the C_4F_8 gas bubble.

Perfluoro-n-butane (C_4F_{10}). Perfluoro-n-butane (C_4F_{10}) is the longest chained perfluorocarbon that can be used intravitreally to tamponade retinal tears. Gases in this group with longer chains exist as a liquid at room temperature. The least soluble perfluorocarbon gas is C_4F_{10}. Experiments in rabbits demonstrated that this gas expands to 5 times the original volume injected, with maximum expansion on the third day. It has a half-life of 20 days. When 0.3 mL was injected intravitreally, the gas completely displaced the vitreous gel in the rabbit. The maximum pressure increase was observed immediately after injection, with return to normal levels within 1 hour.[38]

Wong and Thompson[39] calculated that a maximum of 0.5 to 0.7 mL C_4F_{10} can be injected intravitreally in humans without draining subretinal fluid or evacuating vitreous. Injection of 0.9 mL pure C_4F_{10} produces transient vitreous flare and cell. When the gas was in contact with less than two thirds of the posterior lens capsule, normal lens metabolism continued, preventing the development of cataracts. No retinal toxicity was observed in the rabbits.[38]

TABLE 2–2. GAS COMPOSITION IN VITREOUS AFTER INJECTION OF C_4F_8 *

Hours Postinjection	No. of Eyes	Nitrogen and Oxygen Content (vol%)	Carbon Dioxide Content (vol%)
24	1	97.4	2.6
	2	90.0	10.0
	3	97.3	2.7
	4	91.0	9.0
	5	96.0	4.0
48	1	93.7	6.3
	2	96.4	3.6
	3	97.7	2.3

*Determined by gas-layered chromatography. (From Peyman GA, Vygantas CM, Bennett TO, et al: Octafluorocyclobutane in vitreous and aqueous humor replacement. *Arch Ophthalmol* 1975;93:514–517. Copyright 1975; American Medical Association.)

Perfluoropropane (C_3F_8). Early work by Lincoff et al[40] determined that C_3F_8 stays in the eye 4 times longer than does SF_6. The investigators injected 0.4 cc C_3F_8 into the vitreous cavity of rabbits; maximum expansion was reached on the third day. The gas remained in all rabbit eyes at 25 days and was totally absent by 34 days. Cataracts occurred in all of the eyes (n = 6) because the expanded bubble covered the entire posterior surface of the lens for an extended period. When a second group of rabbits was injected with 0.2 cc C_3F_8, only one of six eyes developed a cataract. The cataracts were thought to be caused by a mechanical interference with transport across the posterior capsule, rather than by a chemical effect of the gas. No discernible retinal damage from the gas was found.[40]

LONGEVITY OF PERFLUOROCARBON GASES

The intraocular longevity of perfluorocarbon gases in human eyes is proportional to the length of the carbon chain. The expected longevity based on intravitreal injection of 1 mL pure gas is 10 to 14 days for SF_6, 30 to 35 days for C_2F_6, and 55 to 65 days for C_3F_8.[35,41] Two milliliters pure CF_4 has a half-life of 6 days and is absent by day 16; 0.8 mL pure C_2F_6 has a half-life of 10 days and completely disappears from the eye after 40 days; the half-life of 1 mL pure C_3F_8 is 35 days, and the gas is absent by 70 days; 0.6 mL pure C_4F_{10} decreases by half the original volume in 45 days and leaves the eye by 120 days.[36]

The insolubility of these gases also increases their expansile properties. Pure SF_6 expands to approximately 2.2 times the volume initially injected, CF_4 to 1.9 times, C_2F_6 to 3.3 times, C_3F_8 to 4 times, and C_4F_{10} to 5 times.[34,40] In animal eyes, CF_4 expanded maximally 1 day after intraocular injection. SF_6 and C_4F_8 demonstrated maximum expansion 2 days after injection, and maximum expansion of C_3F_8 occurred on day 3.[34]

In a study of eyes receiving intraocular concentrations of 15%, 20%, or 25% C_3F_8 in similar clinical settings, Meyers and associates[42] found wide variation in the decay rate and the half-life of this gas. Previous studies have reported significantly different half-lives for 10% C_3F_8 after vitrectomy. A half-life of approximately 30 days was reported by Jacobs et al,[43,44] who calculated intraocular gas concentrations with A-scan ultrasonography. Calculating meniscus height to determine intraocular gas volume, Thompson[45] found the half-life of C_3F_8 to be 5.7 days for phakic eyes, 4.5 for aphakic eyes, and 4.3 for pseudophakic eyes.

The investigators[42] postulate that the difference in method used to calculate intraocular gas volume accounts for some of the variability in decay rate and half-life of C_3F_8 observed in different studies. They noted a prolongation of C_3F_8 in eyes with hypotony. Thompson[45] made a similar observation. In addition, C_3F_8 disappeared more slowly in two patients who were receiving acetazolamide (Diamox, Lederle, Pearl River, NY) and timolol maleate (Timoptic, Merck, Sharp & Dohme, West Point, PA) to control elevated IOP. Delay of absorption in all these eyes was postulated to result from decreased aqueous production.

An additional study[46] included 206 eyes that had undergone pars plana vitrectomy for various vitreoretinal disorders. It demonstrated that the rates of disappearance of various concentrations of C_3F_8 showed a linear regression up to 20% concentration. When gases are required for different periods of intraocular tamponade, it is generally necessary to keep multiple containers of various gases with varied half-lives. This need is obviated by the use of different concentrations of a longer-acting gas such as C_3F_4. The intraocular half-life of air was 1.3 days. It was 4.2 days for 5% C_3F_8, 6.5 for 10%, 8.0 for 15%, and 12.5 for 20%. Mixtures above 12% C_3F_8, 20% SF_6, or 20 to 25% C_2F_8 are intraocularly expansile over a 2-day period.

Lincoff et al[47] noted that diffusion across the retina into the retinal and choroidal circulations is one method of gas removal from the eye. Diffusion of a gas across the retina is inversely proportional to the thickness of the retina. The half-life of perfluorocarbon gas is significantly longer in human than in rabbit eyes. The human retina is 3 times thicker than the rabbit retina.[48,49]

Wong and Thompson[39] found that the duration of a gas bubble is affected by clinical conditions, with the half-life of nonexpansile mixtures of SF_6 and C_3F_8 2 to 3 times greater in phakic rabbit eyes without vitrectomy than in aphakic, vitrectomized rabbit eyes. Reasons for this decreased half-life include trapping of gas in the vitreous gel in phakic eyes, which diminishes absorption of the gas by limiting its intraocular movement. Removal of the lens allows the gas to gain access to the iris and anterior chamber, providing two additional routes of absorption besides the retina and choroid. Finally, convection currents, which in vitro enhance absorption of gases, are created by removal of the lens and vitreous and allow gas to move freely between the anterior chamber and vitreous cavity.

Thompson[45] demonstrated that the half-life of intraocular gases also is longer in phakic than aphakic or pseudophakic human eyes. This study involved injection of air, 10% C_3F_8, and 20% SF_6 after vitrectomy. The half-life of air was 1.6 days in phakic eyes and 0.9 days in aphakic eyes. In eyes receiving 20% SF_6, the half-life was 2.8 days in phakic eyes and 2.4 days in aphakic, and in eyes receiving 10% C_3F_8 it was 5.7 days in phakic, 4.5 days in aphakic, and 4.3 days in pseudophakic eyes.

Lincoff et al[50] intravitreally injected equal amounts of pure CF_4 or C_2F_6 in rabbit eyes. In contrast to Wong and Thompson,[39] they found that the volume of gas in aphakic vitrectomized eyes was 1.3 times greater than that in paired control eyes, demonstrating a prolonged longevity of the expanding gas bubble in eyes after lensectomy and vitrectomy. Comparison of eyes undergoing vitrectomy with control eyes, however, showed no significant difference in the disappearance rate of the expanding gas bubble. These investigators[39] postulate that increased surgical trauma may be partly responsible for the discrepancy in results. Perhaps the most important factor in explaining the different results involves the use of different methods to measure intraocular gas.[39] Wong and Thompson[39] used an indirect method, measuring the height of the meniscus. This technique is prone to error compared with that used by Lincoff et al,[50] where enucleated rabbit eyes were held beneath an inverted funnel and cut open. Gas collected in the funnel was then drawn into a 1-mL pipette and directly measured.[50]

A study by Jacobs et al[44] involved intraocular injection of 12% C_3F_8 and 20%

SF_6 into eyes after vitrectomy as part of a retinal detachment procedure. The 20% SF_6 gas bubble almost immediately began to shrink in size, despite some gas being retained in the eye for up to 2 weeks. With this change in volume over as much as 2 weeks, SF_6 may not be able to provide an adequate internal tamponade to close large retinal tears or breaks located in the inferior retina because the patient may have great difficulty assuming and maintaining an appropriate head posture over such a length of time. In contrast, very little reduction in the size of the C_3F_8 bubble occurred during the first 2 weeks. This provided a very good internal tamponade for large retinal tears and inferior breaks. The bubble may persist within the eye for periods longer than 2 months, with a half-life between 30 and 40 days. Perhaps a nonexpansile mixture of C_2F_6 or C_4F_8 would be better suited as an intraocular tamponade in eyes with proliferative vitreoretinopathy (PVR) because these perfluorocarbon gases have a greater intraocular longevity than SF_6, although they are not as long acting as C_3F_8.

The nonexpansile concentration of C_3F_8 is 12%,[19] and that of SF_6[20] is 20%. In cases of severe PVR, because of the inability to remove all subretinal fluid, a slightly expansile mixture of 20% C_3F_8 is injected intraocularly to ensure a complete intraocular fill while avoiding postoperative glaucoma.[51]

In 1993, the Food and Drug Administration (FDA) approved C_3F_8 and SF_6 for intraocular use in pneumatic retinopexy but not other intraocular uses[52]; Brinton and Hilton[52] note the intraocular use of these two gases for other purposes was not disapproved by the FDA. These investigators further note that two surveys[53,54] involving vitreoretinal surgeons have determined the intraocular use of these two gases, being practically universal, is considered to be the standard of care by these specialists.

DETERMINATION OF INTRAOCULAR GAS VOLUME

The duration of the internal tamponade is determined partly by the kinetics of intraocular gas absorption and the volume of gas inside the eye.[39] Parver and Lincoff[55,56] developed a method of determining the volume of intraocular gas and the area of the retinal wall contacted. Using an emmetropic model eye, they calculated the relationship between volume of gas injected intravitreally and the arc of retinal contact. These investigators found that a 0.28-cm^3 bubble covers 90° of the retina, which is sufficient to tamponade most retinal tears.[55] Significantly greater volumes of gas are required to cover larger tears or similar-sized tears in eyes with axial myopia. Parver and Lincoff calculated that in any eye the volume of gas needed to cover tears of 120° could be determined by multiplying the volume required for a 90° area of bubble–retina contact by 2.7; for a tear of 150°, the multiplication factor was 5.3, and for 180°, 8.6 (Table 2–3). However, their method involved estimating the gas volume through a dilated pupil, and the edges of the bubble's meniscus are difficult to visualize in gas-filled eyes.

A second method of estimating the bubble size involves the use of A-scan ultrasound to detect the volume of intraocular gas or the change in volume of a gas bub-

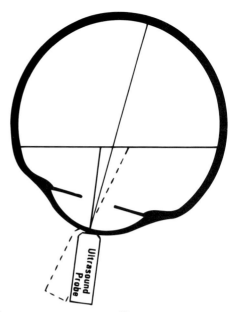

Figure 2–8. Misalignment of eye and ultrasound probe results in underestimation or overestimation of fluid level. (From Jacobs PM: Intraocular gas measurement using A-scan ultrasound. *Curr Eye Res* 1986;5:575–578.)

ble over a specific period (Fig. 2–8).[57] Wong and Thompson[39] developed a third method of estimating bubble size, which uses the height of the bubble's meniscus (parallel to the ground) seen in the plane of the cornea (Fig. 2–9). As an example, a bubble with a meniscus height 40% of the cornea contacts 40% of the retina when the patient is positioned properly.

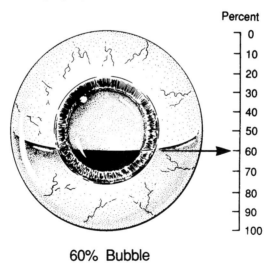

60% Bubble

Figure 2–9. The meniscus height of an intraocular gas bubble is estimated clinically as a percentage of the vertical diameter of the eye seen through the dilated pupil with the plane of the cornea perpendicular to the ground. (From Wong RF, Thompson JT: The prediction of the kinetics of disappearance of sulfur hexafluoride and perfluoropropane intraocular gas bubbles. *Ophthalmology* 1988;95:609–613. Published courtesy of *Ophthalmology* [1988;95:609–13].)

TABLE 2–3. RELATIONSHIP OF BUBBLE VOLUME TO ANGULAR EXTENT (DEGREES) FOR VITREOUS CAVITIES OF VARIOUS DIAMETERS FROM 19 TO 24 mm

Arc of Bubble–Retina Contact (degrees)	Bubble Volume (cm³) for Diameters of					
	19 mm	*20 mm*	*21mm*	*22 mm*	*23 mm*	*24 mm*
90	0.2080	0.2430	0.2800	0.3200	0.3690	0.4200
120	0.5620	0.6560	0.7500	0.8700	0.9900	1.1300
150	1.1100	1.3000	1.4900	1.7300	1.9700	2.2400
180	1.7980	2.1000	2.4000	2.7900	3.1800	3.6200

(From Parver LM, Lincoff H: Mechanics of intraocular gas. Invest Ophthalmol Vis Sci 1978;17:77–79.)

EFFECTS OF INTRAOCULAR GAS ON THE CORNEA

In aphakic eyes, intraocular gases may remain in contact with the corneal endothelium for prolonged periods. A study by Foulks and associates[58] involved intracameral injection of C_3F_8 and SF_6 in cat and rabbit eyes. Clinical and ultrastructural examination showed that both gases resulted in corneal edema, which resolved when the SF_6 bubble reabsorbed. However, corneal edema persisted after the C_3F_8 gas bubble disappeared. Slit-lamp, light, scanning, and transmission electron microscopic examination indicated the presence of corneal edema, endothelial opacities, fibrin deposits, and retrocorneal opacities in corneas exposed to C_3F_8 but not in corneas exposed to SF_6.

Lee and associates[59] studied the toxic effects of gases injected into the anterior chamber of rabbit eyes after paracentesis. Salt solution, sodium hyaluronate, and buffered saline solution (BSS) were considerably less toxic to the cornea and lens than the three gases tested. Fifteen percent C_3F_8 and 50% C_2F_8 were found to be no more toxic than air, whereas 100% C_3F_8 caused considerable toxic effect to the cornea and lens, which was postulated to be caused by the expansile effects of this gas.

Deprivation of aqueous or mechanical contact with the gas is thought to cause the toxic effect on the corneal endothelium, suggesting that longer-acting gases may be more toxic to the endothelium than their shorter-acting counterparts.[59]

EFFECT OF INTRAOCULAR GAS ON THE BLOOD–OCULAR BARRIER

According to Lincoff and colleagues,[34,36,40,60] the perfluorocarbons and SF_6 stimulate a vitreal and preretinal cellular response by altering the blood–retinal barrier.

The effect of intraocular gases on the blood–aqueous barrier is important because breakdown of the barrier may be associated with the intravitreal migration of substances capable of exacerbating PVR.

Ogura and associates,[61] using a fluorophotometric technique, demonstrated that SF_6 and C_3F_8 induced a subclinical breakdown of the blood–retinal barrier after intravitreal injection, resolving on complete reabsorption of these gases. None of the eyes with intravitreal gas demonstrated anterior chamber inflammatory signs when examined with biomicroscopy. Intravitreal air injection failed to have any effect on the blood–retinal barrier.

Results of other studies measuring the integrity of the blood–ocular barrier are contradictory.[62] In the presence of an intravitreal expanding gas bubble of C_3F_8 gas, Sparrow and associates[62] could not demonstrate leakage of intravenously injected gadolinium diethylene triamine penta-acetic acid across the blood–retinal barrier using magnetic resonance imaging (MRI). Wong and Liggett[63] did not demonstrate a measurable inflammatory response in eyes after intravitreal injection of C_3F_8 gas by measuring soluble protein concentration in the vitreous.

Lincoff and colleagues[36] found that approximately 48 hours after intraocular injection of perfluorocarbon gases into eyes without prior vitrectomy, a vitritis reaction developed. Vitreous opacification in rare instances prevented clear visualization of the fundus. Cells and flare remained in the vitreous cavity until the gas totally reabsorbed. Minimal reaction was observed in eyes that had undergone a complete vitrectomy before intraocular gas injection.[36] Animal experiments failed to demonstrate retinal toxicity.[34] Lenticular changes, which occasionally developed in human eyes, were usually reversible after reabsorption of the perfluorocarbon gas.[36]

These researchers suggest that the use of a very-short-acting gas might lessen the uveal response and diminish cellular proliferation when a longer-acting gas is not required.[38] A specific example is scleral buckling, in which a tear is jeopardized by a retinal fold, and the presence of intravitreal gas is needed for only a short time to flatten the fold. Lincoff and Kreissig[64] recommend xenon gas, which is a short-acting inert gas. Ninety percent of xenon disappears from the eye in 16 hours and the remainder within 24 hours of injection. Xenon is able to flatten many retinal folds without providing an excessively long tamponade. A further benefit is a reduction in the amount of time required to position the patient in the presence of intraocular gas.[65]

TECHNIQUE OF INTRAOCULAR GAS INJECTION

The technique used for injection of intravitreal gas (Fig. 2–10) was described by Norton.[25] The importance of avoiding the creation of "fish eggs"—numerous small bubbles that significantly reduce visibility of the retina—cannot be overemphasized. If a bubble is injected into the anterior portion of the vitreous and the needle is placed inside the bubble before additional gas is injected, this results in the creation of one or two large bubbles.

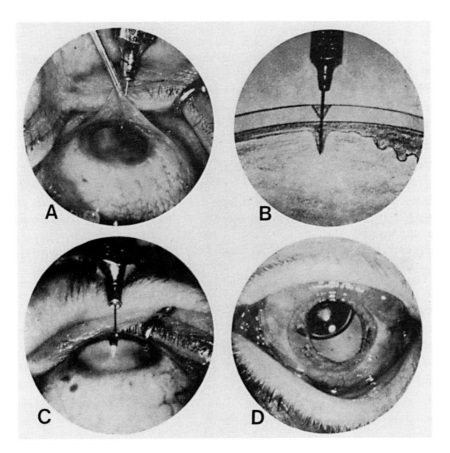

Figure 2–10. Injection of gas into the eye. **A.** Needle pushing ciliary epithelium ahead of tip. **B.** Schematic diagram of needle going into ciliary epithelium. **C.** Needle tip free in vitreous cavity. **D.** Single gas bubble in vitreous cavity. (From Norton EWD: Intraocular gas in the management of selected retinal detachments. *Trans Am Acad Ophthalmol Otolaryngol* 1973;77:OP85–OP98.)

Gas minifies the retinal image when viewed with an indirect ophthalmoscope. We find visibility best with a 28-diopter (D) hand-held lens.

Precautions must be followed in patients given intravitreal injections of inert gas. Nitrous oxide (N_2O) should not be used as a general anesthetic when gas is injected intraocularly into the closed eye.[66] If already in use, the use of N_2O should be discontinued up to 20 minutes[66,67] before intraocular injection of a gas bubble, which allows depletion of N_2O through the respiratory system, lowering tissue concentrations of this gas.[66,68,69] Otherwise, N_2O has been shown to cause rapid expansion of an intraocular gas bubble,[66,67,70] which can cause significant elevation of IOP in the eye of an individual receiving N_2O anesthesia.[66,67,71] Postoperatively, a rapid reduction in the gas bubble volume may occur after the use of N_2O anesthesia.[67]

Changes in atmospheric pressure also cause expansion of the gas. We advise patients who have intraocular gas not to fly in airplanes as long as gas is present because doing so may precipitate an acute attack of glaucoma.[72] Eyes with intraocular gas lose the insulating capacity of a normal eye, and cryopexy must be done more gently and with a smaller ice ball to avoid overfreezing the retina.

The use of an intraocular gas in vitrectomy surgery is widespread. Excess intraocular gas from an expanding bubble may cause significantly elevated IOP, which, if undetected, can result in visual loss from a central retinal artery occlusion.

When attempting a complete fill of the posterior chamber with an expanding gas bubble, caution must be exercised. If the posterior chamber completely fills, the anterior segment becomes shallow and IOP rapidly rises. Adequate lowering of IOP can only be achieved by removing gas from the posterior segment.[44] However, elevated IOP after retinal detachment surgery also has been reported when photoreceptor outer segments block the trabecular[73,74] meshwork, when patients have preexisting primary open-angle glaucoma,[75,76] and when the surgery has caused decreased aqueous outflow.[75,76]

In a series of 30 patients injected with one of four perfluorocarbon gases, pressure increased abruptly to between 35 and 50 mm Hg, but returned to normal (20s) within 90 minutes.[36] Subretinal fluid was not usually drained before intraocular injection. Providing the central retinal artery was patent, the investigators believed the elevated pressure was not a cause for concern. The few eyes with sustained pressure elevations responded to medication or paracentesis. Several eyes were prophylactically treated with acetazolamide and timolol maleate.[36]

INTRAOCULAR GAS AND INTRAOCULAR PRESSURE

The degree of efficiency of topical beta-blockers and carbonic anhydrase inhibitors in lowering IOP in gas-filled eyes is unknown. Therefore, at times, aspiration of fluid or gas is used to reduce IOP. A study by Simone and Whitacre[75] demonstrated that an identical reduction in IOP is produced by removing an equivalent volume of gas or fluid.

The accuracy of various tonometers in measuring IOP in gas-filled or air-filled eyes varies considerably. Goldmann applanation tonometry provides the most accurate values, but its use may be limited by postoperative lid edema, by corneal epithelial or other surface defects, by fluorescein, or by marked astigmatism. Postoperative difficulties in patients and the lack of portability are disadvantages to using the Goldmann applanation tonometer.[77]

Traditional methods of measuring IOP in normal eyes may give inaccurate readings in the gas-filled eye. Schiotz tonometry is unreliable because the retinal detachment surgery and pressure of a compressible intraocular gas reduce scleral rigidity.[78] This form of tonometry was found to underestimate the IOP when compared with manometric readings in gas-filled enucleated eyes.[78] In gas-filled vitrectomized eyes with corneal edema, applanation tonometry also underestimates IOP.[79,80] Unlike the Goldmann applanation and Schiotz tonometers, the MacKay-Marg tonometer accurately measures IOP in eyes with irregular corneas caused by surgery, edema, or scarring.[81,82] The Tono-Pen (Menton O & O, Norwell, MA) (Fig. 2–11), a small, hand-held device that does not require a slit lamp, measures IOP. It has been demonstrated to be as accurate as the MacKay-Marg in measuring IOP in eyes with irregular corneas after epikeratophakia and keratoplasty and in scarred corneas.[83] A plunger surrounded by a larger front plate is placed against the cornea. The force generated by the plunger activates a strain gauge; pressure first increases and then is relieved by the front plate. This change is recognized by a microprocessor chip and, after several small, pecking movements by the operator, several measurements are averaged and a digital reading is given.[84-87]

In a study[88] of 47 eyes after pars plana vitrectomy and gas–fluid exchange at pressures greater than 25 mm Hg, no significant differences were detected between the Tono-Pen and the Goldmann tonometer. The Tono-Pen, in general, demonstrates a small tendency to overestimate IOP. Other studies confirm that this portable tonometer may be useful in measuring IOP after vitrectomy.[77,84,86,88-90] In contrast, in gas-filled eyes, pneumatic tonometry tended to underestimate IOPs significantly.[73] An additional study involving a small number of eyes with intravitreal gas demonstrated that the pneumatic tonometer may underestimate IOP by more than 5 mm Hg.[91]

A regression curve for the vitrectomized air-filled eyes that represents manometric readings has been developed for the Tono-Pen. By referring to this curve, any Tono-Pen reading in an air-filled eye can be translated into the corresponding manometric reading.[92] Lim et al[93] failed to show any correlation between IOP and the size of the intraocular gas bubble. These investigators conducted a clinical and a manometric study involving human eye bank eyes, comparing Tono-Pen and pneumotonometer readings with manometric IOP.

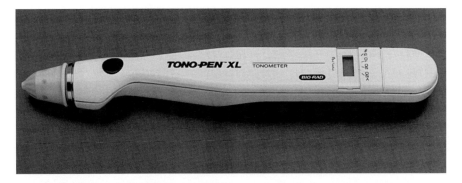

Figure 2–11. Tono-Pen XL. (Courtesy of Mentor O & O, Norwell, MA.)

Based on data from these experiments, the investigators[93] concluded that both tonometers significantly underestimated IOP when IOP was greater than or equal to 25 mm Hg. At IOPs in the lower 20s mm Hg, the readings from the pneumotonometer and Tono-Pen correlated with the true IOP. To evaluate the real IOP, the investigators provided conversion tables to avoid underestimating IOP in vitrectomized gas-filled eyes, especially in the presence of glaucoma or retinal vascular disease, in which failure to detect a highly elevated pressure can cause serious complications.

When possible, we use applanation tonometry to determine IOP in air- or gas-filled eyes. IOP is checked immediately after the procedure, at 6, 12, and 24 hours after the gas exchange, and then daily if there has not been a significant increase in IOP, until the gas has had the opportunity to reach maximum expansion. If expansile mixtures have been used and IOP is measured above 30 mm Hg by applanation tonometry, a 30-gauge needle attached to a tuberculin syringe is placed through the limbus in aphakic eyes or the pars plana in phakic eyes, and a small volume of gas is withdrawn. When some fluid is present inside the eye, removal of fluid may be preferred.[94]

VOLUME OF THE INTRAOCULAR GAS BUBBLE

Lincoff and associates[95] have used expanding perfluorocarbon gases injected intravitreally, without draining subretinal fluid or removing vitreous, to tamponade posterior retinal tears temporarily. This approach is used when treatment by conventional techniques would be difficult and would compromise final visual acuities. After retinopexy with either cryocoagulation or argon laser coagulation, the maximal adhesive strength of the lesion takes 9 to 11 days to develop.[95,96] To be effective, a volume of gas sufficient to tamponade the tear must remain in the eye for a minimum of 9 days.

These researchers[95] determined that a gas volume of 1 mL was sufficient to cover most posterior tears. Injection of 0.6 mL C_3F_6, which expands by a factor of 3.3, can usually be carried out without draining subretinal fluid if ocular massage is performed. This amount of gas provides a 1-mL intravitreal gas bubble on the ninth day. Many patients are unable to remain in a prone position for 5 days. A volume of 2.4 mL effectively covers the macular area when the patient assumes any position.

Han and associates[97] compared the effect of two concentrations of perfluoropropane gas considered to be nonexpansile (12%) or slightly expansile (20%) in a randomized prospective study involving 30 nonglaucomatous eyes undergoing pars plana vitrectomy for complicated retinal detachment. No statistical difference between the groups was observed in postoperative IOP, bubble size at 36 to 48 hours, and final IOP. In contrast, the duration of the intraocular tamponade was longer in the 20% group. The mean duration to complete the disappearance of the bubble and the duration of time to a 50% fill was longer in the 20% group compared with the 12% group (8.4 versus 6.7 weeks, and 3.5 versus 2.4, respectively).

RETINAL FOLDS AFTER GAS INJECTION

Twomey and Leaver[98] reported the development of large, flat retinal folds in 10 eyes after successful repair of rhegmatogenous retinal detachment. They had used a circumferential retinal buckle, drainage of subretinal fluid, and intraocular gas as an internal tamponade. The retinal folds were radially oriented, originating either from the posterior aspect of the buckle or optic nerve; in three cases they involved the macula.

These investigators[98] postulated that an encircling scleral buckle caused a reduction in the circumference of the inner eye wall in relation to the underlying detached retina. Redundant retina is created in the meridian corresponding to the long axis of the exoplant. Consequently, the retina demonstrates circumferential redundancy, which is proportional to the height, width, and length of the buckle while being relatively shortened in the anterior–posterior meridian.

Lewen et al[99] reported three eyes with superior rhegmatogenous retinal detachments in which a circumferential scleral buckle and intravitreal air injection were associated with the formation of acute retinal folds. These unusual retinal folds arose from the end of a hard silicone exoplant. Vision is compromised when the acute folds involve the macula. Excessive tightening of the encircling buckle in eyes without intravitreal gas will by itself also produce retinal folds.

Posterior Retinal Folds

Larrison and associates[100] described posterior retinal folds occurring in 28 eyes after vitrectomy, air–fluid exchange, and scleral buckling and four eyes with scleral buckling surgery combined with intraocular gas injection. The investigators postulate that, after drainage of fluid through a peripheral retinal break in eyes with partial retinal attachment, residual retinal fluid accumulates posteriorly in a dependent position. Fluid that is also forced posteriorly is sequestered at the dependent posterior margin of the retinal detachment that is located at the attached/detached retinal border. The elevated retina assumes the appearance of a retinal fold in this location as the RPE pumps out the residual fluid. Posterior retinal folds are significant when the macula is involved, causing metamorphopsia and decreased vision. Drainage of subretinal fluid through a posterior retinotomy with complete removal of subretinal fluid may prevent this complication.

DISPLACEMENT OF SUBRETINAL FLUID AFTER GAS INJECTION

Postoperatively, subretinal fluid can be displaced in the presence of a large gas bubble. The rapid reabsorption of the fluid causes the redundant retina either to fold on itself or be compressed by the bubble. Avoidance of a large gas bubble may prevent significant posterior displacement of subretinal fluid, which increases the risk of detaching the macula.

STORAGE OF GAS

Humayun et al[101] measured the rate of diffusion of SF_6 from a capped plastic syringe (10 cc) that is commonly used to inject that gas into an eye. Using gas chromatography at 30 seconds, the concentration was 97%; at 15 minutes, 89%; at 60 minutes, 76%; and at 18 hours, 2%. The investigators postulated that the gas escaped across the porous plastic walls of the syringe and that the rate of gas loss from a capped syringe with a 30-gauge needle probably would be similar. The investigators noted that marked differences in the concentrations of intraocularly injected SF_6 occur with changes in interval between aspirating the gas and intraocular injections. Very accurate ratios of both gas and air concentrations are necessary to calculate the exact intravitreal bubble size and duration necessary to provide an accurate intraocular tamponade. To ensure accurate concentrations of SF_6, the gas should be aspirated just before anticipated intravitreal injection.

In contrast to results with SF_6, a report by Cummings et al[102] noted that C_3F_8 concentrations were stable for up to 120 minutes after aspiration into plastic syringes. Raymond and associates[103] performed experiments measuring the air content over a 12-month period of 30-mL plastic syringes filled with instrument-grade C_3F_8 (98%). Three months after filling, the air content had increased to 25%. The investigators noted that pure C_3F_8 stored for up to 3 months in plastic syringes can be used for intraocular injection; the gas has predictable expansile properties that allow the surgeon to compensate for the decreased expansile ability of the gas by increasing the volume of injected gas.

Storage of SF_6 Gas in Vacutainer

Friedrichsen and associates[104,105] demonstrated that SF_6 gas can easily be stored in 10-mL Vacutainer tubes (Becton Dickson Vacutainer System, Rutherford, NJ), which provide a back-up source of gas should the gas be needed in an area remote from where the cylinder is stored. The tubes must be free from an anticoagulant coating or any particulate material. A residual air volume of 2.7 mL (± 0.15) was present in all tubes supplied from Becton Dickson Vacutainer Systems. A 27-gauge needle attached to a syringe filled with pure SF_6 was allowed to equalize with the Vacutainer tube. The filled tubes contained 81% SF_6 with a standard deviation of 0.8% when the procedure was performed at sea-level barometric pressure and normal room temperature. Higher concentrations of SF_6 would be present at greater elevations because the air in each tube is constant, and the equalizing pressure of SF_6 varies depending on the altitude. No change in gas concentration was demonstrated over a 3-month period.

Removal of SF_6 is accomplished by injecting into the tube an amount of balanced saline solution (maximum, 5 mL before seal is lost) equivalent to the amount of gas to be withdrawn, which briefly pressurizes the tube.

All procedures included in gas storage and withdrawal are performed using a Millipore filter (Millipore Corp., Bedford, MA). To obtain the required concentration of gas, the SF_6 removed from the tube is mixed with air. At sea level, a 4-to-1 dilution is required to obtain a 20% SF_6/air mixture.[104,105]

AIR–FLUID EXCHANGE

Air–Fluid Exchange in an Operating Room Setting

Air or gas is used intraoperatively after vitrectomy. It tamponades the retina against the RPE and allows the formation of chorioretinal adhesions after laser, diathermy, or cryopexy (Fig. 2–12).[44,106,107] The high surface tension of gases assists in closing retinal tears (Fig. 2–13), and the buoyancy of the gas bubble allows it to conform to the margins of irregular retinal tears.[106]

The air–tissue interface closes the retinal hole. It decreases the flow of fluid from the vitreous cavity through the hole, permitting the RPE and choroid to reabsorb the subretinal fluid, resulting in reattachment of the retina.

Tiny retinal breaks visible preoperatively by fundus biomicroscopy may be difficult to locate during vitrectomy. These breaks can be marked with argon blue-green laser using a small spot size and moderately high energy.[108] Application of transvitreal diathermy to the retina before fluid–gas exchange ensures visualization of breaks during gas–fluid exchange. Excessive diathermy should be avoided to prevent formation of a retinal break.[109]

Air enters the eye through an infusion cannula (Fig. 2–14), which is connected to the air pump. Generally, the infusion line for irrigation solution and air tubes are connected by a tri-stopcock to the infusion cannula sutured at the pars plana site.

An illuminated switch can precisely indicate whether the air or infusion fluid line is open. Because the system is independent from the room illumination, the operating room nurse can activate the air or the infusion fluid line by pressing the switch without disturbing the dark adaptation of the surgeon.[110]

Air–fluid exchange can be combined[110] with internal drainage of subretinal fluid (Fig. 2–15). The pressure of the air pump is set at approximately 50 mm Hg. The air pump maintains the IOP automatically by increasing the flow of the air inside the eye despite the leakage of any air through the sclerotomies. Air enters the eye through the infusion cannula while aspiration of fluid in the anterior vitreous cavity is performed with either a fluted needle or an extrusion handpiece. The blunt or tapered needle, called an extrusion handpiece, is usually connected by a polyethylene tube to the vitrectomy console, which provides vacuum. The needle is vented externally through an opening on the body of the instrument similar to some disposable vitreous suction cutter handpieces.[111] Aspiration of fluid vitreous or subretinal

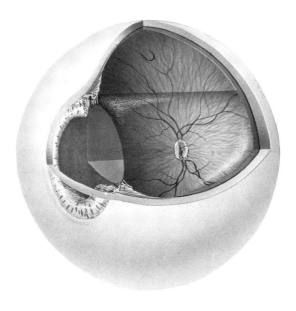

A

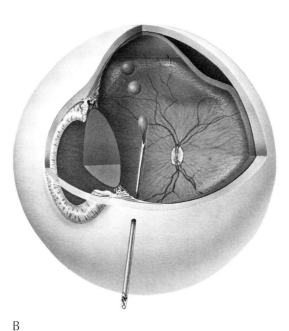

B

Figure 2–12. **A.** Schematic representation of a localized retinal detachment with a retinal tear. **B.** Air or gas is injected in the eye to provide a tamponade. **C.** The patient is positioned to achieve absorption of subretinal fluid. **D** and **E** (page 80). Laser coagulation of tear is performed to create a chorioretinal scar.

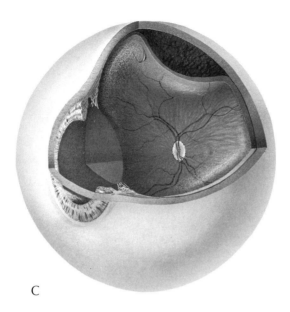

C

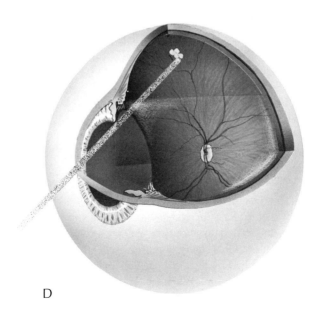

D

Figure 2–12 (Continued).

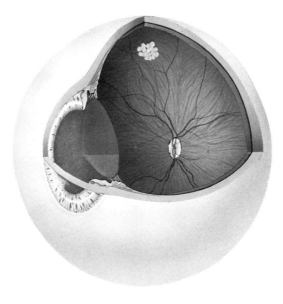

E

Figure 2–12 (Continued).

fluid is performed when suction is applied to the tube and the operator's index finger is used to close the aperture on the body of the instrument. When the aperture is opened, air is sucked into the system, and the suction becomes discontinuous. If the suction line is completely clamped, the suction needle functions like a flute needle.[112] In such a situation, the IOP forces the fluid from the vitreous cavity through the needle and out of the opening on the handle of the instrument.[113]

Oftentimes, multiple bubbles that coalesce initially enter the eye. The needle is then gradually moved toward the posterior pole when a posterior retinal tear is present or toward a prepared retinotomy site. Subretinal fluid is pushed posteriorly as the air–fluid exchange progresses[114] and is evacuated using a flute needle.[115]

Drainage of subretinal fluid through a retinotomy can be performed with an extrusion cannula, which is blunt tipped, tapered, or has a soft silicone tip or extension.[116] The cannula, attached to an automated suction, is placed slightly anterior to the retinal hole until the subretinal fluid is almost completely removed. At this point, a meniscus of fluid is touched by the cannula. This maneuver is repeated until re-attachment of the retina has occurred. When the fluid falls below the level of the cannula tip, a bright reflex is observed as the needle touches the fluid and the reflex disappears, which helps avoid direct contact between the needle tip and RPE. The positive pressure created by the infusion of gas and controlled linear suction applied to the cannula results in the removal of subretinal fluid through the suction needle (Fig. 2–15).[114]

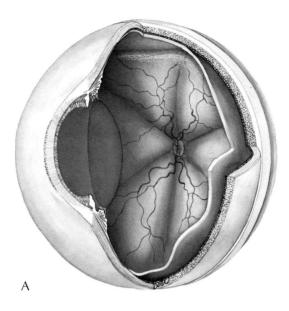

A

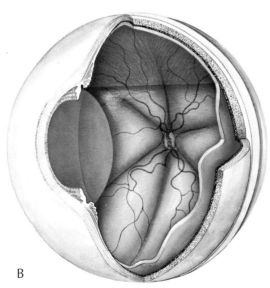

B

Figure 2–13. Technique to localize suspected retinal tear with intraocular gas. **A.** Injection of perfluorocarbon gas in the vitreous cavity. **B** and **C.** Retinal detachment persists until the gas bubble reaches below the level of the retinal tear in **D. E** (page 83). When gas is reabsorbed, the gas bubble rises above the retinal tear, and the retinal detachment reappears.

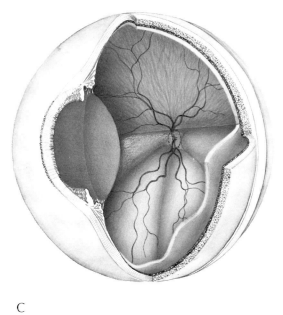

C

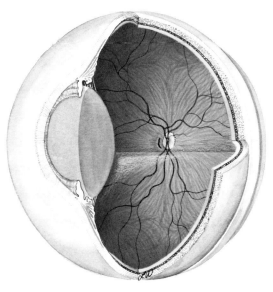

D

Figure 2–13 (Continued).

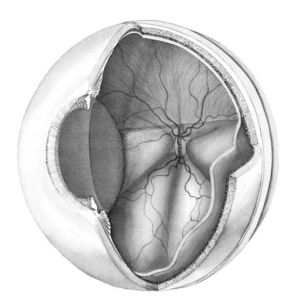

E

Figure 2–13 (Continued).

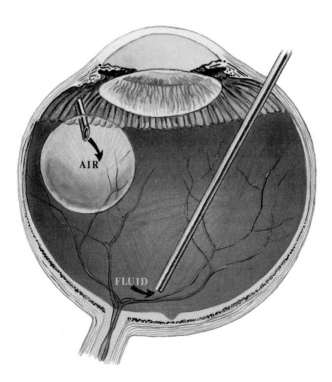

Figure 2–14. Graphic representation of air–fluid exchange.

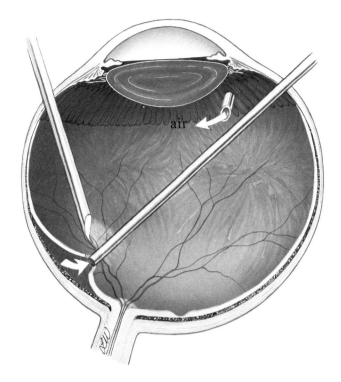

Figure 2–15. Air–fluid exchange and internal drainage of subretinal fluid.

The retina must be carefully observed during the air–fluid exchange and the internal drainage of subretinal fluid. When areas of epiretinal traction exist, forceful air injection may cause existing tears to enlarge or may create large tears at the site of preexisting traction.

Failure of the retina to flatten or the presence of subretinal air indicates residual traction that must be relieved before the retina will reattach. Subretinal air may not easily be removed because it can migrate anteriorly.

Air–fluid exchange in many cases allows assessment of the effectiveness of intraoperative surgical techniques in relieving retinal traction. During air–fluid exchange, residual areas of traction become identifiable.

A multitude of intraocular manipulations can be accomplished in an air-filled eye to relieve residual retinal traction, including creation of a relaxing retinotomy and epiretinal membrane dissection and segmentation.

When performed intraoperatively in eyes with PVR, air–fluid exchange can indicate the location and extent of additional membranes. These areas generally tent up and necessitate further membrane dissection to obtain retinal reattachment.[107]

Air–fluid exchange in the presence of an intraocular lens (IOL) can be complicated by the anterior displacement of the IOL against the cornea. Diddie and Smith[117] recommend the initial placement of two 27-gauge needles through the clear cornea. A bolus of gas is injected into the anterior chamber, which replaces aqueous that is passively being drained by the second needle. The gas–fluid exchange is performed in the usual manner. The composition of the gas injected into the anterior chamber and vitreous cavity should be the same. The gas in the anterior chamber prevents forward movement of the pseudophakos.

Several techniques have been used to create a drainage retinotomy,[114] including the use of the vitreous suction cutter to create a retinal hole.[113] This retinal hole may have irregular edges, may be larger than required, or may be associated with retinal hemorrhage. A retinal perforator was developed by Gonvers to cut through retina, but again bleeding may occur from severed retinal vessels.[118] A third method is to use a microvitreoretinal (MVR) or similar blade to cut detached retina, which is often difficult; it can make the retinotomy size difficult to control and, like the other methods, is associated at times with retinal bleeding.[115] To avoid these complications, a unipolar cautery with either a blunt or tapered tip has been developed to create a small round hole with a white rim when applied against elevated retina. The possibility of hemorrhage is avoided by the cauterization of retinal vessels.[114]

Failure of the diathermized necrotic retina to perforate occasionally necessitates the use of a sharp blade or suction needle to accomplish the task.[118]

Evacuation/cautery needles have been developed that combine cautery with passive suction. They allow clearing of any vitreous hemorrhage overlying the retinotomy site and cauterization of underlying bleeding vessels without interchanging instruments (Fig. 2–16).[119,120] These instruments also permit creation of a retinotomy and internal drainage of subretinal fluid to be performed with the same instrument.

Retinotomy sites used to be created at the superior nasal or inferior nasal side of the optic disc. Because complications are associated with drainage of subretinal fluid, these sites may be in the superior 180° of the retina, where air or silicone tamponade is facilitated.[121] Manipulation of the eye can place even relatively anterior drainage sites in a position that allows adequate subretinal fluid drainage without the use of soft silicone extrusion tubing.[122]

Complications using a standard stainless steel flute needle to drain subretinal fluid include retinal incarceration, possible enlargement of the retinotomy site, and retinal or subretinal hemorrhage. A tapered extrusion needle lessens the likelihood of this complication, and a back-flush needle allows incarcerated tissue to be freed.[114,116] The retina around the drainage site must be almost totally devoid of subretinal fluid to allow laser treatment in the area. The flute needle may inadvertently touch the underlying RPE as the retina becomes almost attached, damaging both the RPE and underlying Bruch's membrane and resulting in choroidal bleeding. Late complications at the retinotomy site from this damage include subretinal neovascularization and the formation of preretinal and subretinal tractional retinal detachment. Reopening of the endodrainage sites as a result of local proliferation causes recurrent retinal detachment. When surgery is necessary to relieve traction, this proliferative tissue requires excision at the retinotomy site before its removal can be completed.[122]

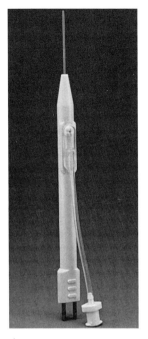

A

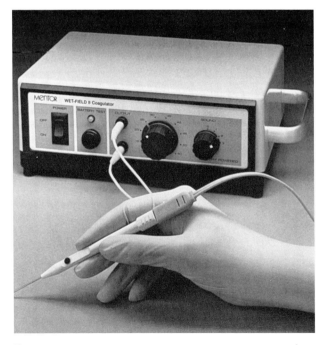

B

A

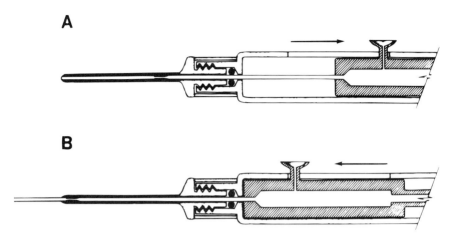

B

Figure 2–17. Schematic drawing of the cannulated extrusion needle. **A.** The slide mechanism is shown retracted, bringing the flexible tubing within the metallic 20-gauge needle shaft. Note the safety features of the instrument, including the snug fit of the cannula inside the 20-gauge needle, the O-ring seal at the base of the needle, and the outer seal surrounding the screw fit. **B.** The slide mechanism is shown in advanced position. The flexible tubing is extended for up to 18 mm beyond the rigid tip. The distal end of the handpiece can be connected to a syringe or to the vitrectomy console for active suction if the surgeon covers the venting hole with an index finger. (From Flynn HW, Lee WG, Parel J-M: Design features and surgical use of a cannulated extrusion needle. *Graefes Arch Clin Exp Ophthalmol* 1989;227:304–308.)

The use of a silicone-tipped needle may lessen the damage created during internal drainage of subretinal fluid. To avoid complications at the retinotomy sites, trauma must be minimized while internally draining subretinal fluid, which can be accomplished by keeping the flute needle above or at the level of the retinotomy site. Care should be taken to avoid excessive thermal damage to Bruch's membrane during endophotocoagulation to achieve chorioretinal adhesions.[122]

A cannulated extrusion needle[114,123-125] has recently been developed (Fig. 2–17). A flexible 24-gauge silicone cannula is attached to a tapered metal tip that can be extended 18 mm by moving a slide control. When a venting hole is open, passive egress of fluid from the eye occurs. Alternatively, active suction can be applied by connecting the needle to the vitrectomy console with tubing and covering the venting hole.

The primary use of the cannulated extrusion needle has been to drain subretinal fluid internally through the existing tear, without the need to create a retinotomy in eyes with complicated retinal detachment associated with PVR (Fig. 2–18).[114,124]

Figure 2–16. A. Disposable intraocular aspiration probe with bipolar cautery and reflux capabilities. **B.** Mentor Wet-Field II Coagulator with disposable evacuation/cautery needle. (Courtesy of Mentor, Inc., Norwell, MA)

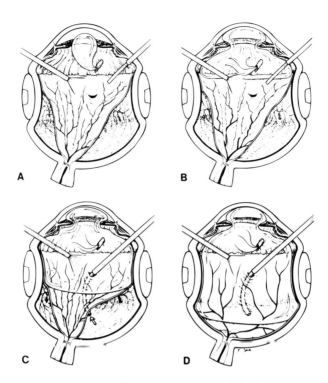

Figure 2–18. Surgical technique for internal subretinal fluid drainage in a PVR case with a scleral buckle in place. **A.** Air enters the eye by way of the sutured pars plana infusion cannula, assisted by the automated air pump. Fluid in the vitreous cavity leaves the eye through the flexible cannula as the air bubbles fill the anterior portion of the globe. **B.** The flexible cannula is guided into the peripheral retinal break as soon as the multiple air bubbles in the anterior portion of the globe begin to coalesce. The enlarging air bubble pushes the subretinal fluid posteriorly. **C.** The external venting hole is open to allow the positive pressure of the continuous air pump to push the subretinal fluid out of the external venting hole. **D.** The retina is reattached overlying the subretinal cannula. The venting hole is again covered, and the flexible cannula is retracted into the shaft of the rigid extrusion needle before the removal of the instrument from the pars plana sclerotomy. (From Flynn HW, Lee WG, Parel J-M: Design features and surgical use of a cannulated extrusion needle. *Graefes Arch Clin Exp Ophthalmol* 1989;227: 304–308.)

Initially, as air enters the eye, fluid in the vitreous cavity is removed either passively or with active suction using the cannulated extrusion needle. The flexible cannula is then guided into the subretinal space through a peripheral retinal break and directed obliquely into the area containing the highest elevation of posterior subretinal fluid, with care being taken not to direct the cannula into the macular area, because tracks can occur there. Subretinal fluid then can be removed using passive egress or active suction. The tip should be placed parallel to the RPE to remove subretinal fluid most effectively.[114,124]

Other advantages of the cannula include the ability to observe the flow of sub-retinal fluid to determine whether the internal drainage process is proceeding adequately. The smaller 24-gauge tip, as compared with a standard 20-gauge tip, lowers the risk of retinal incarceration by permitting a more controlled flow of subretinal fluid. This fluid is removed more slowly than with the use of rigid instrumentation held over a retinotomy site or retinal hole but does not require the repeated pauses needed to allow additional subretinal fluid to collect over the retinal drainage site. The flexible silicone tubing should also minimize the risk of bleeding when the choroid or retina is touched.[114,124]

Additionally, vitreous hemorrhage, subretinal fluid, and residual fluid that are difficult to remove by other techniques can be readily aspirated in the subretinal space with the cannulated extrusion needle.[114,124]

Other uses for this system include the removal of preretinal blood using the vacuum-cleaning technique[126] and the collection of fairly pure samples of subretinal fluid.[114]

Occasionally a layered hyphema appears somewhat adherent to the retina and is difficult to remove. The ability to touch the retina atraumatically with this instrument permits removal of this preretinal blood.

In most cases in one series,[114] after subretinal placement, a hypopigmented track developed corresponding to the subretinal path of the cannula, but no instances of subretinal hemorrhage caused by the cannula were documented. One patient developed intraretinal hemorrhages attributed to the cannula, which resolved within a few weeks and did not lead to any hole formation.

The cannulated extrusion needle may also be used in selected giant tears to unroll the edges of the giant tear with the patient in a supine position while a fluid–gas exchange is performed with an automated air pump. The retina can be picked up using suction and can also be pulled anteriorly with the cannulated extrusion handpiece.[114,125] Additional uses of this instrument include the removal of subretinal silicone and gas[114] and drainage of subretinal hemorrhage involving the macula and caused by macular degeneration or complications of a previous retinal detachment.

Air–Fluid Exchange in an Outpatient Setting

Air–fluid exchange in an outpatient setting after vitrectomy is indicated for recurrent vitreous hemorrhage to remove intravitreal blood. This procedure facilitates retinal examination and is an alternative to vitreous washout, which involves a second surgery. Removal of intraocular blood with replacement by air or an air–gas mixture facilitates visualization of any retinal pathology, allows management of possible complications, prevents unnecessary delay in visual recovery, and may protect against rebleeding in some instances. This procedure is also useful in persistent or recurrent retinal detachment to close retinal breaks by providing an internal tamponade. It allows subretinal fluid to be absorbed and laser photocoagulation to be applied to the retina surrounding the breaks. A chorioretinal scar can develop in the treated area, which more securely attaches the retina to the underlying pigment epithelium. The intraocular presence of a long-acting gas in PVR also allows the retina more time to become adherent to the pigment epithelium.[94,127,128]

Stern and Blumenkranz[129] advise using a 20% mixture of SF$_6$ and air. Two milliliters pure SF$_6$ are placed in a 10-mL syringe. Using sterile tubing, connections, and a 0.22-μm Millipore filter attached to the gas tank to ensure sterility, 8 mL air is withdrawn into the syringe to provide the desired concentration of gas. Gas is then expelled from the syringe until 5 mL remains. Patients are placed in a prone position in bed with the chin supported by a pillow. After topical anesthesia, a wire lid speculum is placed in the patient's eye. Using light from either an indirect ophthalmoscope or a flashlight held by an assistant, the surgeon stabilizes the eye with a cotton-tipped applicator, and air–fluid exchange is done through the limbus in aphakic patients.

We have found that patient stability and surgical control are achieved by using the slit-lamp chin rest to support the head. The slit-lamp light beam is used to illuminate the eye. Two Tylenol (acetaminophen; McNeil, Fort Washington, PA) No. 3 tablets are given 30 minutes before the procedure to reduce or eliminate ocular discomfort. After the application of topical anesthesia and before the procedure, the cul-de-sac is irrigated first with a 10% povidone-iodine (Betadine, Purdue Fredricks, Norwalk, CT) solution and then with sterile BSS. A drop of topical gentamicin is placed on the cornea, and the eye is entered through the temporal limbus with a 27-gauge, 0.714-inch needle attached to the syringe (Figs. 2–19, 2–20). Before it enters the eye, the needle is beveled to prevent escape of intraocular gas and the production of hypotony when it is withdrawn from the eye.

The needle is placed slightly below the pupil, fluid is withdrawn, and gas is injected in 0.3-mL increments. Wide variations of IOP must be avoided to prevent severe ocular pain. Fluid collects in the bottom of the syringe. When the anterior chamber begins to fill with gas, the needle is moved inferiorly, and additional fluid is withdrawn and replaced with air. When the eye is filled with gas, the needle is withdrawn. If hypotony is present at the end of the procedure, the IOP is reestablished by injecting a 20% mixture of SF$_6$ and air through the limbus with a 30-gauge, 0.5-inch needle in aphakic patients. The same procedure is performed through the pars plana in phakic eyes.

Retrobulbar anesthesia is used to perform this procedure in phakic eyes. The patient is placed in a prone position in bed, with the head tilted toward the side of the involved eye. After insertion of the lid speculum, the needle is inserted through the temporal pars plana 4 mm behind the limbus. When the needle is visualized behind the lens, the exchange is started. The needle is gradually retracted as gas accumulates in the vitreous cavity. The procedure is terminated when air is withdrawn from the syringe. After the procedure, IOP is measured by applanation tonometry. A drop of gentamicin is placed on the eye, and the IOP is recorded 4 to 6 hours later and again the next morning.[129]

Variations of this technique have been described. The needle on the syringe can be placed through the temporal limbus in aphakic eyes or the pars plana in phakic eyes.[94] Positioning of the patient may vary during this procedure.[94,127] The patient may be placed in a face-down position in bed or on a stretcher with the head resting on the arms, which are folded across a pillow.

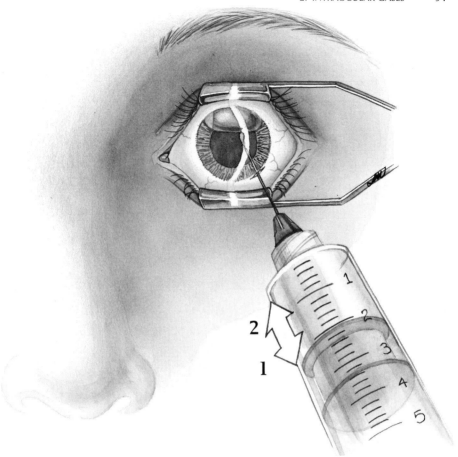

Figure 2–19. Schematic representation of outpatient air–fluid exchange through the limbus using a syringe. Arrow indicates back-and-forth motion of the piston for withdrawal of fluid and injection of gas.

Eyes treated with techniques that rely on injection of gas followed by fluid withdrawal in sequential cycles tend to experience the accumulation of multiple small bubbles ("fish eggs"). This occurs when the gas moves to the most superior position in the eye. These fish eggs can take 24 hours to resolve; initially they prevent fundus visualization. A way to avoid fish eggs is to position the needle so that the tip is inside the gas bubble as injection continues (Fig. 2–21). This causes the bubble to enlarge with additional gas but is only applicable when two needles are used, one for injection of gas and the other for withdrawal of fluid. Maneuvering the needle intraocularly to place the tip within the preexisting bubble may result in inadvertent contact between the needle and the lens.[94]

The technique for performing outpatient air–fluid exchange has been modified to involve the use of two syringes to prevent formation of fish eggs and overinfla-

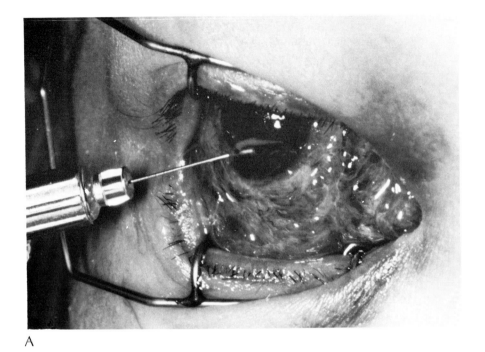

A

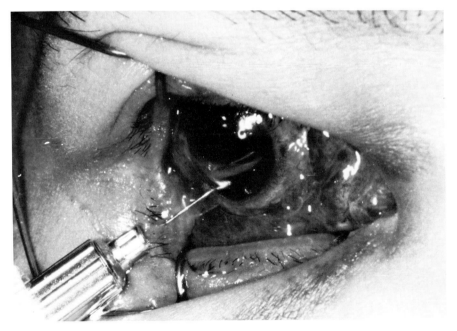

B

Figure 2–20. Photographs of gas–fluid exchange. **A.** The needle is placed in the anterior chamber. **B.** Two-thirds exchange is done. **C.** Gas–fluid exchange is completed.

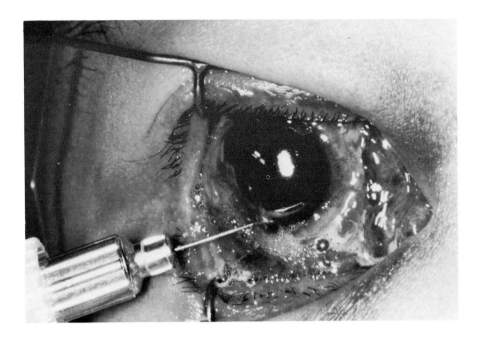

C

Figure 2–20 (Continued).

tion of the globe. After retrobulbar anesthesia, Miller and associates[130] place the patient in a horizontal position with the eye undergoing exchange in a more dependent position. A 26- or 27-gauge, 0.625-inch needle attached to a syringe is placed through the temporal pars plana by the surgeon. A second needle is inserted, which is connected by sterile tubing to an air–fluid pump with the pressure output setting adjusted to approximately 25 mm Hg. This needle is placed through the pars plana, away from the lens, along the horizontal meridian on the nasal side. The air pump is turned on while the surgeon simultaneously aspirates fluid from the vitreous cavity and allows a single large air bubble to form inside the eye while the eye maintains a constant pressure; this is in contrast to the overinflation and repetitive collapse of the globe that occurs with the single-needle technique. When all fluid has been removed from the eye, the needle through the temporal pars plana is removed, followed by withdrawal of the needle connected to the air pump. This technique requires two trained ophthalmologists.

Another similar technique that allows the intraocular injection of gases has been described.[131] Using extension tubing, a three-way stopcock is attached to an air pump. The stopcock is adjusted to allow air to flow into the eye from the air pump, which is turned on with the pressure set at 40 mm Hg while the second syringe aspirates vitreous fluid. When a complete exchange has been performed, the stopcock is turned so that gas from the 35-mL syringe can be injected into the eye. This tech-

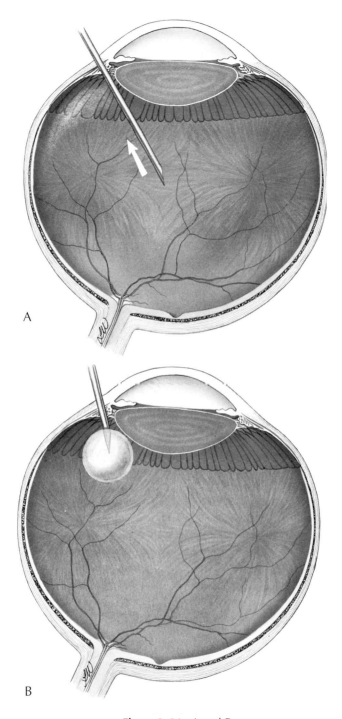

Figure 2–21. A and **B.**

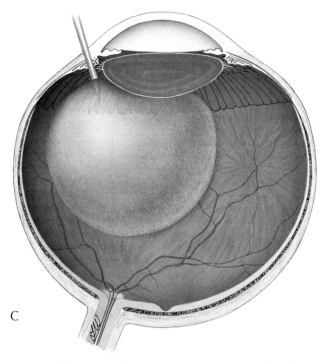

C

Figure 2–21. A. A needle connected to an air syringe is inserted in the eye; the tip of the needle is visible through the pupil, then the needle is retracted slightly (arrow). **B.** The needle is retracted, and air is injected slowly. **C.** The rest of the air is injected in the air bubble to prevent fish egg formation.

nique allows air to be removed from the eye while a mixture of 20% C_3F_8 or 25% SF_6 is injected. A nonexpansile gas–air mixture is formed inside the eye. Long-acting gases are not advised in phakic eyes because prolonged lens contact can cause a cataract.

A new instrument for performing fluid–gas exchanges consists of two small stainless steel tubes. Use of this instrument minimizes surgical fatigue and is especially valuable in phakic eyes, where contact between the lens and needle may accidentally result in cataract formation.[132]

At the end of the procedure, after withdrawal of a needle, we usually apply a cotton swab with gentamicin ointment to the needle tract to prevent escape of intraocular gas, and topical gentamicin drops are applied after the procedure is finished. When the needle is placed through the limbus, the needle tract is shelved so that on removal it tends to be self-sealing. Replacement of a needle after premature withdrawal before the procedure is finished should be done through a separate site because insertion through the initial tract may stretch this opening and result in subsequent leaks.[94] When iris becomes incarcerated in the inner cornea, gentle massage with a blunt instrument over the external cornea in the area of the incarceration usually releases the tissue.[90] When removing blood, a 30-gauge needle may become obstructed, and a 25-gauge needle creates too large a tract in the cornea, which may subsequently leak and make use of a 27-gauge needle preferable.[90]

In addition to wound leak and iris incarceration, other potential complications during gas–fluid exchange include bleeding from contact between the needle tip and iris, corneal endothelial injury, cataract caused when the needle touches the lens, choroidal effusion, central retinal artery occlusion associated with intravitreal injection of an expansile gas, and (rarely reported) endophthalmitis.[94,133] Glaucoma can occur from early expansion of an intraocular gas, raising IOP or causing pupillary block glaucoma in aphakic patients when the gas bubble blocks the pupillary aperture.[133]

Before intraocular injection of an expansile gas, gonioscopy should be performed to detect eyes with compromised angles, which may have areas of closure caused by peripheral anterior synechiae or neovascularization. Only nonexpansile gases should be used in these eyes, and all patients with a significant gas fill should be advised to assume a face-down position to avoid aphakic pupillary-block glaucoma, angle-closure glaucoma, and lenticular opacities.[128] Concentration of 12% to 14% C_3F_8, 15% perfluoroethane (C_2F_6),[128] and 18% to 20% SF_6[127] have been found to be nonexpansile.

When possible, we use applanation tonometry to determine IOP in air- or gas-filled eyes. IOP is checked immediately after the procedure; at 6, 12, and 24 hours after the exchange, and then daily until maximum expansion of the gas can occur if expansile mixtures are used. If IOP becomes elevated above 30 mm Hg as measured by applanation tonometry despite initiation of maximal medical therapy, a 30-gauge needle attached to a TB syringe is placed through the limbus in aphakic eyes and pars plana in phakic eyes, and a small volume of gas is withdrawn. When some fluid is also present inside the eye, its removal may be preferable.[94]

FLYING AND INTRAOCULAR GASES

Many vitreoretinal surgeons use perfluorocarbon and other gases as an adjunct to vitrectomy,[53] and their patients are often discharged from the hospital shortly after surgery. The first-order exponential absorption of many of these gases allows gas bubbles in some instances to remain in the eye for long periods.[47] Lincoff and associates[47] determined that a patient with a residual gas volume of 0.6 mL, which represents approximately 10% of the eye, can safely withstand a decompression produced at 8,000 feet above sea level during ascent of an aircraft without a corresponding dangerous elevation in IOP. Larger intraocular gas bubbles can be tolerated safely if decompression of a plane is at a lower level than 8,000 feet above sea level.[134]

Previous instances of vision loss and ocular pain occurring during ascent of an airplane[134,135] have prompted investigators to evaluate the effect of cabin decompression on the expansion of an intraocular gas bubble and IOP.[72,134-138]

Lincoff and associates[137] documented in rabbit eyes that gas bubbles occupying as much as 10% of the total intraocular volume could adjust to a simulated decrease in cabin pressure corresponding to 8,000 feet over 27 minutes with a small IOP increase of 6 mm Hg despite an expansion of 34%, which was compensated for by accelerated aqueous outflow, choroidal compression, and scleral expansion. In a survey of airline pilots and aircraft manufacturers, the investigators learned that 8,000 feet as a standard for compression was a maximum and rarely reached. In actuality, most aircraft decompress to less than 8,000 feet after reaching cruising altitude. The usual time taken for an airplane to decompress cabin pressure to 8,000 feet is 27 minutes.[138]

A patient with intraocular gas who experiences ocular pain or decreased vision should request that the pilot descend to the next flight level to reduce cabin pressure by approximately 1,500 to 2,000 feet, which will lower IOP by approximately 50% and probably relieve symptoms. Should symptoms persist, the pilot could be asked to reduce altitude by one more flight level, which would require FAA approval. The investigators also found that the prophylactic use of preflight medications such as timolol maleate or acetazolamide sodium lowers IOP insignificantly. After descent and landing, such medications can cause ocular hypotony, and choroidal effusion can develop. Prophylactic breathing of 100% O_2 had no effect on the volume of the intraocular bubble.[138]

PNEUMATIC RETINOPEXY

Dominguez,[139] Hilton and Grizzard,[140] Boyd,[141] and Tornambe[142] have used expansive intraocular gases instead of scleral buckling to treat patients with rhegmatogenous retinal detachments on an outpatient basis.

Indications for Pneumatic Retinopexy

Hilton et al[143] reported on a series of 100 patients that included cases with aphakia, pseudophakia, macular breaks, trauma, old retinal detachments, vitreal hemorrhage, and macular detachment. Eyes with PVR grades C and D and mentally incompetent patients were excluded from this study.

Indications for pneumatic retinopexy have expanded considerably. Several series[142,144,145] have reported good anatomic results in eyes with more complex retinal detachments. Pneumatic retinopexy was successful in treating four eyes with multiple retinal breaks located more than 30° apart. Kamp-Mortensen and Sjolie[144] treated 12 patients with retinal tears located superiorly between the 8 and 4 o'clock positions. Pneumatic retinopexy was successful in reattaching the retina in 10 eyes after the initial procedure. Tornambe et al[146] reported on a series of 40 eyes in 39 patients with multiple breaks in different quadrants and up to 6 clock-hours apart, retinal detachments associated with moderate degrees of PVR not exceeding grade C_2, large tears up to 2.5 clock-hours in size, and inferior breaks. In eyes with multiple breaks, the patient was initially positioned to close the most superior break and then repositioned after 1 to 2 days to close the inferior breaks. When breaks were nearly equidistant from the 12 o'clock meridian, the patient was rotated every 4 hours to cover each break alternately. Positioning was maintained for 5 days, and all breaks did not have to be simultaneously closed.[146]

Pneumatic retinopexy may be used to repair a recurrent detachment after scleral buckling procedures. A buckled eye is less rigid than an unbuckled one, so that there is diminished risk of significant elevation of IOP at the time of gas injection.[147] After retinal reattachment, cryotherapy either cannot treat a retinal tear through a silicone buckle, or can do so only with great difficulty, and treatment of breaks posterior to the buckle requires a conjunctival incision.

Additionally, intraocular gas may be used in surgery in conjunction with scleral buckling to prevent hypotony after drainage of subretinal fluid, or to minimize residual traction or flatten retinal folds that may result at times in "fishmouthing" of a retinal tear. In the immediate postoperative period, intraocular gas may be injected to tamponade a previously unrecognized retinal tear. This approach may be used to flatten retinal folds or to treat a suspected but not visualized tear if the retina has failed to reattach.

Pneumatic Retinopexy Technique

The surgical procedure involves the intravitreal injection of an expansile gas in conjunction with the sealing of the retinal break by laser photocoagulation or cryocoagulation. The retina can be reattached by using the gas to bring the sensory retina in contact with the RPE. The inflammatory reaction induced by laser energy or cryocoagulation seals the retinal hole.

This procedure is limited to retinal detachments caused by retinal breaks in the superior half of the retina, mainly between the 8 and 4 o'clock positions. Patients with widely separated tears (two or more holes 60° or more apart) and those who have inferiorly located holes are not considered ideal candidates for this surgery. Other contraindications are the presence of glaucoma, PVR, and iris-supported or anterior chamber IOLs and patients who cannot comply with postoperative orders because of physical or mental problems. The patient's cooperation is important to achieve and maintain the tamponading effect of the gas bubble (Fig. 2–22).

Pneumatic retinopexy appears to offer several advantages over conventional scleral buckling surgery: ambulatory management of retinal detachment, reduced patient discomfort and surgical costs, less tissue manipulation, and avoidance of refractive changes and motility disorders associated with scleral buckling. The procedure can be performed in an examination room in the office or an outpatient minor surgery room.

Preoperatively, Hilton and Grizzard[140] dilate the pupil. Topical anesthesia is

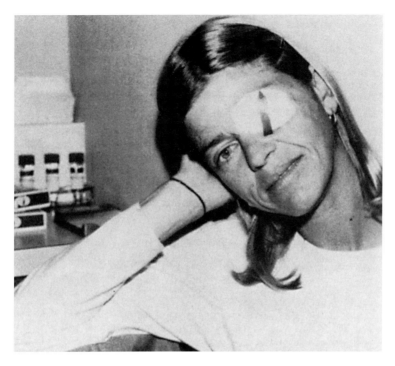

Figure 2–22. The meridian of the retinal break is marked on the bandage with colored tape or a felt-tipped pen. With the periodic use of a hand mirror, the patient can easily position the head by pointing the arrow toward the ceiling. (From Hilton GF, Grizzard WS: Pneumatic retinopexy: A two step outpatient operation without conjunctival incision. *Ophthalmology* 1986;93:626–641. Published courtesy of *Ophthalmology* [1986; 93:626–41].)

used in aphakic eyes, whereas phakic eyes require retrobulbar anesthesia. Anesthesia is followed by the use of oral osmotic agents, a Honan IOP reducer, digital massage, or a combination of these methods to reduce IOP.

Transconjunctival cryopexy is applied contiguously around the break. Pressure applied to the globe during this procedure may be adequate to reduce the IOP without the use of the previously mentioned adjunct means of lowering IOP. A wire eyelid speculum is used during gas injection, and the conjunctiva is treated with a few drops of a solution consisting of betadine and an equal amount of balanced salt. Generally, 0.3 mL C_3F_8 or 0.6 mL SF_6 is withdrawn from a tank using a Millipore filter and injected using a 30-gauge, 0.5-inch needle placed through the uppermost pars plana in an area away from the highly elevated retina. Frequently, the patient is placed in a supine position with the head rotated 45° to the side before injection. A sterile, cotton-tipped applicator is used to cover the injection site after the needle is withdrawn, and the head is positioned so that the bubble is away from the injection site. The central retinal artery is observed intermittently for 60 minutes using indi-

rect ophthalmoscopy. If the artery is closed for 10 minutes in the absence of spontaneous pulsations, IOP is lowered in phakic eyes by anterior chamber paracentesis
and in aphakic or pseudophakic eyes with a ruptured posterior capsule by vitreous
aspiration. IOP is also monitored by applanation tonometry for 60 minutes (Fig.
2–23) followed by instillation of an antibiotic drop and placement of an eyepad over
the eye. Diamox (Lederle, Pearle River, NY), 250 mg, is administered 4 times a day
for 3 days if the patient lives in or intends to visit an area where the altitude is above
4,000 feet. After injection, the head is positioned so that the gas bubble tamponades
the tear, and the patient is instructed to maintain this position for 16 hours a day. The
set positioning is maintained for 5 days. Follow-up examinations are scheduled on
postoperative days 1 through 3, and then 1, 2, 4, 8, 16, and 26 weeks after surgery.
If needed, additional laser or cryopexy is performed during these visits. Two weeks
after surgery, the patient may return to work.

In the presence of a bullous retinal detachment or when subretinal fluid threat-
ens to detach the macula, a steamroller technique is used[146] (Fig. 2–24). The intravitreal gas bubble is positioned at the macula, which forces subretinal fluid away from

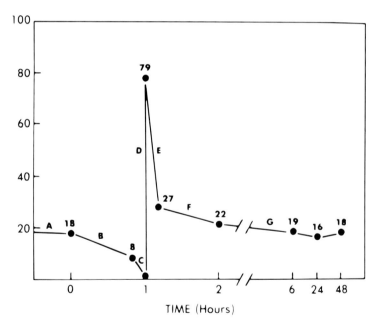

TIME (Hours)

Figure 2–23. **A.** IOP is within normal limits. **B.** The pressure is reduced with the Honan
balloon and oral isosorbide. **C.** The IOP is further reduced, to zero, with pressure from
the cryoprobe. **D.** The IOP is elevated by the injection of gas. **E.** The IOP typically
remains normal after the first hour. (From Hilton GF, Grizzard WS: Pneumatic
retinopexy: A two step outpatient operation without conjunctival incision. *Ophthalmology* 1986;93:626–641. Published courtesy of *Ophthalmology* [1986;93:626–41].)

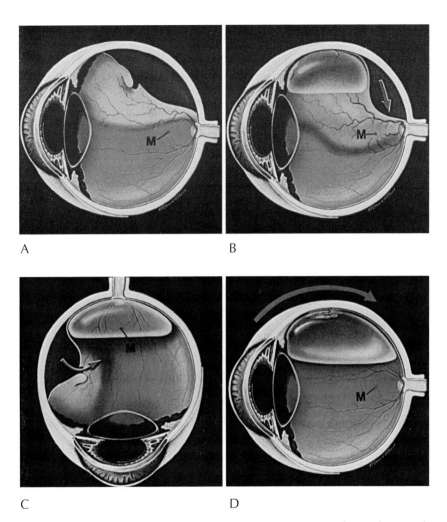

A   B

C   D

Figure 2–24. A. Bullous retinal detachment adjacent to a normal macula. **B.** Infrequently, the gas bubble may force fluid posteriorly, causing detachment of the macula. **C.** The potential problem of iatrogenic macular detachment (**B**) may be prevented by immediately placing the patient in a face-down position so that the bubble flattens the macula. This frequently causes subretinal fluid to pass through the break into the vitreous (arrow). **D.** The position of the patient's head is slowly moved through a series of incremental changes, along the meridian between the macula and the retinal break. This movement requires 20 to 30 minutes, resulting in placement of the retinal break uppermost. The subretinal fluid is usually forced into the vitreous by the steamroller effect of the slowly moving bubble. (From Hilton GF, Kelly NE, Salzano TC, et al: Pneumatic retinopexy: A collaborative report of the first 100 cases. *Ophthalmology* 1987;94:307–312. Published courtesy of *Ophthalmology* [1987;94:307–12].)

this area. Over a short period (approximately 20 minutes), the head is shifted so the tear is placed in the uppermost position; this forces fluid out of the tear and into the vitreous, causing the retina to flatten. Because this technique may force RPE cells from the subretinal space into the vitreous cavity, retinal cryopexy is not performed until the retina around the tear flattens.[148]

The technique used for pneumatic retinopexy has been modified. The patient is placed in a supine position and the head turned to one side. The needle is inserted in an area away from highly elevated retina and withdrawn so only 2 to 3 mm remains inside the eye. When performing a vitreous tap or aqueous tap in aphakic eyes or eyes with a ruptured posterior capsule, the needle is inserted through the pars plana to avoid vitreous incarceration, which may be associated with a limbal paracentesis.[149] When C_3F_8 is used, 0.3 to 0.8 mL pure gas is injected. When less than 0.5 mL of gas is injected, elevation of IOP is rarely a problem.[149]

Instead of preoperative application of cryopexy around the tear, subretinal fluid is allowed to reabsorb, then laser photocoagulation is applied around the break. Experimental evidence suggests that a permanent adhesion is formed faster by laser than by cryopexy. The laser adhesion forms shortly after treatment.[150]

Gunnerson and associates[151] additionally drained subretinal fluid in eyes with highly elevated detachment. Retinal elevation interferes with the ability to perform cryopexy.

When tears are multiple and the angle of gas coverage must be increased, gas injections may be repeated daily or even more frequently. The volume of gas necessary to cover all tears can be calculated from the experiments performed by Parver,[152] which determined the size of a gas bubble required to cover different angles of the retina.[152] After withdrawal of the needle after gas injection, a cotton-tipped applicator covered with a large amount of antibiotic ointment is placed over the scleral needle track and the eye rotated to move the bubble away from the injection site to prevent loss of intraocular gas. Postinjection, the patient is placed on timolol maleate eye drops twice a day.

In the presence of multiple retinal breaks in different quadrants, the patient's head position can either be changed at 4-hour intervals or the superior breaks treated initially for a few days, followed by repositioning of the head to treat inferior breaks.

The binocular indirect ophthalmoscope laser delivery system[153] has been used to perform laser coagulation after pneumatic retinopexy. This system provides several benefits to the surgeon performing this procedure, including the ability to apply treatment to the ora serrata (with the aid of scleral depression); to place laser treatment on the scleral buckle; and to easily visualize the retina around a gas bubble. The patient's head can be moved to position the bubble in a way that exposes different areas of the retina during photocoagulation.[20,147,153,154] By reducing RPE cell dispersion, laser photocoagulation theoretically also minimizes the risk of PVR development.[155]

We usually treat retinal tears with laser photocoagulation,[155] using the slit lamp or indirect ophthalmoscope delivery systems.

Contraindications to Pneumatic Retinopexy

Ocular contraindications to pneumatic retinopexy include retinal detachment associated with significant vitreoretinal pathology, such as lattice degeneration, fixed folds, significant vitreoretinal traction, giant tear, or present or previous surgery for giant tear in the contralateral eye. Physical conditions that may limit patient positioning, such as arthritis, mental retardation, and medical conditions, including asthma and congestive heart failure, may preclude pneumatic retinopexy.

Results of Pneumatic Retinopexy

Recently, reports have questioned the success rate of pneumatic retinopexy when compared with the high success rate of scleral buckling procedures, which have been successful in reattaching 76% to 96% of uncomplicated retinal detachments.[156-158] Results from 26 series on pneumatic retinopexy, involving 1,274 eyes, demonstrated that 80% of eyes were reattached after one procedure, whereas 98% were reattached with reoperations.[159]

In a series reported by Tornambe et al,[146] 30 eyes (75%) were successfully attached with pneumatic retinopexy, and the rate increased to 83% if eyes were excluded that had inferior tears in the lower one third of the fundus that could not be effectively treated with pneumatic retinopexy. Eight eyes that underwent conventional retinal detachment surgery were reattached, giving a total anatomic success rate of 95%. Aphakic and pseudophakic eyes had a lower reattachment rate than phakic eyes.

In a prospective series of 51 patients with a 6-month follow-up, Chen et al[156] reported success rates for pneumatic retinopexy of 63% in phakic eyes, 74% in aphakic eyes, and 41% in pseudophakic eyes. McAllister et al[157] compared in a retrospective study uncomplicated cases of retinal detachment treated with pneumatic retinopexy (n = 56), a Lincoff balloon (n = 28), and a scleral buckling procedure (n = 78). After a follow-up period of at least 6 months for all eyes, the reattachment rate was 71% for eyes treated with pneumatic retinopexy, 64% for eyes treated with a Lincoff balloon, and 96% for those treated with an encircling scleral buckle. The incidence of new tears in these groups was 20%, 18%, and 1.3%, respectively. Pneumatic retinopexy was successful in only 43% of aphakic or pseudophakic patients with a ruptured posterior capsule, whereas the rate of anatomic retinal reattachment was 81% in these eyes when the posterior capsule was intact.

Requirements for successful treatment of retinal detachments in the past have included detection and permanent closure of all retinal tears and relief or reduction of vitreous traction.

Complications of Pneumatic Retinopexy

Retinal Tear. Several reports document a fairly high incidence of new or undetected retinal tears, especially in aphakic or pseudophakic eyes after pneumatic retinopexy.[156,157,159-165] A 21% incidence of new breaks was reported by the

Pneumatic Retinopexy Multicenter Clinical Trial.[164] The breaks were more common in pseudophakic and aphakic eyes; most breaks were reported within the first month after surgery.[164] These tears may be either breaks not detected preoperatively or new retinal breaks caused by transmitted vitreous traction. Displacement of vitreous by gas injection, gas expansion, or movement of gas can cause acute vitreoretinal traction.[166] Alternatively, some retinal tears may be extremely small. Similar tears were not detected preoperatively in 16% of aphakic eyes.[166] In another study, investigators[167] reported a 14% incidence in retinal breaks occurring in eyes that had been treated for retinal breaks with intravitreal gas injection and laser photocoagulation or cryopexy, or a combination of both techniques.

Uemura[168] reported a series of 72 eyes with superior rhegmatogenous retinal detachments treated with scleral buckling, with and without intraocular gas. Five eyes developed new retinal breaks postoperatively. Factors associated with the postoperative development of a retinal detachment included the use of a large volume of injected gas, and the presence of intraocular adhesions. Distortion of the vitreous gel resulting in traction in areas of vitreoretinal adhesion immediately after intraocular injection of large volumes of gas was postulated to result in the development of the new retinal detachment.

Dreyer[160] noted that new inferior tears frequently result from the shifting of intraocular gas superiorly, with subsequent vitreous traction greatest 180° from the gas bubble, which is in the area of the interior vitreous base.

PVR. Previous studies of pneumatic retinopexy have reported that the incidences of PVR and premacular membranes vary from between 3%[149] and 5%[169] to 2%[156] and 4%.[170] Use of cryopexy or laser photocoagulation after the retina has flattened may limit the dispersion of RPE cells, which predispose to PVR.[149] Expanding long-acting gases have been demonstrated to induce structural[170,171] and biochemical[36] changes in the vitreous and to alter vitreous protein and cellular content.[36,172] These factors after retinal detachment appear to predispose an eye to develop PVR. Lincoff et al[170] demonstrated shrinking and tearing of the cortical lamellae in monkey eyes, which was produced by an expanding C_2F_6 gas bubble, with some edges displaying early membrane formation by 6 weeks. Progressive biochemical or cellular activity is suggested by the delay of vitreous organization until the gas reabsorbed. The vitreous disturbances described in these studies[36,170-172] may result in the opening of preexisting breaks or creation of iatrogenic tears, in some instances leading to retinal detachments.[149] The probable tractional contraction and separation of the posterior cortical membrane and vitreous resulting from expansion and movement of the gas bubble also may cause these results.

In an attempt to reduce the incidence of PVR and preretinal membrane formation, Sebag and Tang[173] performed a pneumatic retinopexy with air. Their study was composed of 45 eyes with single or multiple retinal tears within 3 clock-hours of each other and with breaks located between 8:00 and 4:00. A stab incision with a 30-gauge needle in the inferior temporal quadrant was performed, followed by a slow injection of 0.8 mL filtered air. During injection, the needle tip was visualized with indirect ophthalmoscopy. All eyes required paracentesis. A second paracentesis was performed in some eyes when the central retinal artery pulsated after 10 minutes. Initial reattachment was achieved in 86.7% of eyes (39), with secondary scleral buckling surgery required in the remaining six eyes to achieve retinal detachment. Visual acuity was the same or better in 97.9% of eyes (n = 44). PVR developed in one case (2.2%), and an additional eye (2.2%) demonstrated a premacular membrane. New or missed retinal breaks were found in 8.8% (four eyes).

Bochow et al[35] noted that perfluorocarbons may be advantageous when performing pneumatic retinopexy compared with SF_6. As a result of increased expansion, a smaller amount of perfluorocarbon gas is required for initial injection, frequently resulting in a lower initial increase in IOP. The lower solubility of the perfluorocarbon gases may result in a prolonged intraocular tamponade, facilitating chorioretinal adhesions because of increased persistence of the perfluorocarbon gas, which maintains closure of the retinal breaks.

Bochow et al[35] used 0.25 to 0.5 mL pure C_2F_6 in 17 eyes with single retinal breaks or groups of breaks no greater than 1 clock-hour. These breaks were located in the 6 superior retinal clock-hours between 9 and 3 o'clock. This perfluorocarbon was selected because of an intermediate duration of action between SF_6 and C_3F_8 and greater expansion of C_2F_6 compared with SF_6. After the initial procedure, 71% (12 eyes) were attached. The remaining five eyes required two or three procedures to achieve retinal reattachment. The investigators postulated that the smaller volume of C_2F_6 required for injection (compared with SF_6) would result in fewer new holes forming postoperatively because of diminished vitreoretinal traction. Fewer paracenteses would be required. At follow-up after 6 months, two eyes (12%) were found with postoperative PVR, one (6%) with premacular fibroplasia, none with cataracts, and three (18%) with new or missed holes. Vision was the same or improved in nine eyes (100%) with preoperatively attached maculas and in seven of eight (88%) with detached maculas. These investigators conceded that further studies are necessary to determine if C_2F_6 has any advantage over other commonly used intravitreal gases when used for pneumatic retinopexy.

SUBRETINAL GAS

Subretinal gas (fish eggs) can be observed after intravitreal gas injection. Entry into the subretinal space through a retinal break is probably facilitated by the presence of numerous small gas bubbles. This complication may be prevented by tapping the globe gently, which usually causes the small bubbles to coalesce into a larger bubble. If subretinal gas is observed despite these precautions, the patient should be positioned so the bubble may escape through the retinal break.[153,174]

McDonald et al[174] reported the presence of subretinal gas after pneumatic retinopexy in seven patients. Head positioning allowing the subretinal gas to enter the vitreous cavity was successful in three patients. Three other eyes required vitrectomy with air–fluid exchange, whereas the remaining eye was treated by closing the retinal tear, despite the subretinal gas, using conventional scleral buckling.

Subretinal gas migration in all cases followed intravitreal injection of multiple small gas bubbles. Injection of a single gas bubble should avoid this complication. Techniques to minimize intravitreal injection of multiple bubbles include positioning the patient so the injection site is at the most superior position of the eye, placement of the needle tip in the anterior vitreous just in front of the pars plana, and rapid injection of the gas bolus. When multiple bubbles are injected, a cotton-tipped applicator can be bent and allowed to recoil against the sclera next to the bubble, which often results in coalescence of the gas into one large bubble.

Wong and associates[175] postulate that intraocular gas, before becoming subretinal, must reach the retrohyaloid space by either direct injection or through holes in the posterior hyaloid, where traction on the anterior retinal tear opens retinal breaks. Alternatively, unrelieved vitreoretinal traction may open retinal breaks and facilitate passage of gas into the subretinal space. Prevention of this complication is possible by using a scleral implant to close the retinal holes. These investigators[175] also note that positioning is not helpful in the treatment of subretinal gas. Pars plana vitrectomy combined with air–fluid exchange is recommended instead for treating this complication.

OTHER COMPLICATIONS OF INTRAOCULAR GAS INJECTION

Other complications reported after pneumatic retinopexy include extension of retinal detachments,[176] macular hole, macular puncture,[159] opening of previously closed tears,[156] never-closed retinal breaks,[159] delayed reabsorption of subretinal fluid, endophthalmitis, cataract, and mild uveitis.[177]

Subretinal pigment migration has been reported after pneumatic retinopexy. This complication is correlated with the amount of cryopexy, vitreous pigment, or "tobacco dust," which may be reduced by minimizing the intensity and number of cryopexy applications.

Infrequently reported complications include choroidal detachment,[159] uveitis,[159] vitreous loss,[159] gas entrapment between the pars plana and the lens,[159] and endophthalmitis.[149,159,164] Application of several drops of 10% Betadine (Purdue Frederick, Norwalk, CT) solution for 3 minutes to the conjunctiva usually prevents this complication.[159,178-180]

Additional operative complications of pneumatic retinopexy include vitreous incarceration at the pars plana injection site,[158] central retinal artery occlusion,[150] vitreous hemorrhage[150] (which usually occurs at the pars plana injection site), gas in the anterior hyaloid space, subretinal gas,[150] subconjunctival gas,[151,177,181] vitreous loss through the needle tract,[177] pars plana pigment epithelial detachment when injection is attempted in an area of elevated pars plana,[169,181] malignant glaucoma,[177] iris incarceration,[177] anterior chamber lens touch, and subretinal hemorrhage.[177] Vitreous hemorrhage and subretinal hemorrhage have been attributed to fracturing of frozen blood vessels caused by movement of a cryoprobe.[164]

In one eye, a cataract developed because of accidental injection of the lens during paracentesis.[159]

Malignant glaucoma was reported in one patient, who ignored instructions and failed to remain prone, thus allowing the gas bubble to cause blockage at the plane of the ciliary body and divert aqueous posteriorly.[159]

Injection of Gas in Retrolental Space

Two cases were reported in which gas was inadvertently injected behind the lens in front of the anterior hyaloid membrane, which assumed an arcuate configuration.[181] Failure to remove gas from this potential space between the anterior hyaloid face and lens could have resulted in a retinal dialysis, a dislocated lens, or cataract caused by gas expansion. Causes of injection of gas in this space may have included an unusually tough anterior hyaloid capsule, excessive withdrawal of the needle into this space after insertion in an attempt to prevent fish eggs, or the use of a dull needle tip. Treatment involves gas removal by inserting a 30-gauge needle vented to the atmosphere into the pars plana over the gas bubble, followed by injection of a second gas bubble.[181]

If the needle tip fails to enter the vitreous cavity or the injection is in an area of elevated pars plana epithelium, sub–pars plana gas may result. Treatment of large elevations involves the use of a plungerless syringe with a 25-gauge needle. The needle is inserted through the pars plana to allow the gas to escape.[149]

CLINICAL TRIAL OF PNEUMATIC RETINOPEXY VERSUS SCLERAL BUCKLING

A multicenter randomized controlled clinical trial involving 198 patients with rhegmatogenous retinal detachments compared pneumatic retinopexy with scleral buckling.[164] To be eligible, tears could not be located within the inferior 4 clock-hours of the fundus, with breaks not exceeding 1 clock-hour in size. Groups of breaks had to be located within 1 clock-hour of each other. Eyes with advanced PVR exceeding grade C_3 were ineligible. All eyes were followed for at least 6 months after surgery.[164]

Reattachment rates after a single operation were 82% for scleral buckling and 63% for pneumatic retinopexy. Reattachment rates for one operation and use of postoperative laser or cryopexy were 64% and 81%,[164] whereas the overall rates for final anatomic success with all operations were 98% at 6 months[164] and 99% at 2 years. Despite the method of treatment, similar anatomic results were achieved with phakic and aphakic/pseudophakic eyes, with the latter group having lower retinal reattachment rates regardless of whether scleral buckling or pneumatic retinopexy was used. Most aphakic/pseudophakic eyes that required reoperations had successful retinal reattachment when scleral buckling was performed. In eyes in which the macula had been detached preoperatively for 14 days or less, a final visual acuity of 20/50 or better was present at the 6-month follow-up in 56% of eyes that underwent scleral buckling and in 80% of eyes treated with pneumatic retinopexy; and by 24 months this acuity was found in 67% of eyes that had received scleral buckling and 89% of those treated with pneumatic retinopexy. If the macula had been detached longer than 2 weeks before surgery, both groups had similar visual results at 6 months; if the macula had been attached at the time of surgery, similar visual acuities were achieved at 6 and 24 months.[149,164] Additionally, vision was restored more rapidly in the pneumatic retinopexy group. More eyes in the scleral buckle group than in the pneumatic retinopexy group had a visual acuity of 20/100 or worse 1 month postoperatively. New or missed breaks occurred more frequently in the pneumatic retinopexy group compared with the scleral buckling group (23% versus 13%). The presence of a new break in the pneumatic retinopexy group did not usually affect the final outcome, with 23 of these 24 eyes (95%) ultimately being reattached and 20 eyes achieving a final visual acuity of 20/50 or better.

Most breaks occurred within the first month after surgery, suggesting that a retinal detachment is unlikely to occur in an eye that has remained reattached for 3 months after surgery.[149,164]

Eyes with breaks that were discovered after initial scleral buckling procedures had a poor eventual outcome, with ultimate reattachment achieved in 83% and a visual acuity of 20/50 or better in 33% of eyes. As a group, these eyes also required more extensive surgical procedures.[164]

The 24-month study found that only a single eye (at 11 months) in the scleral buckling group developed a break after 6 months. This finding indicates that an eye in this group that remained attached for 6 months was unlikely to detach.[149]

Proliferative vitreoretinopathy and macular pucker evolved with similar frequency in both groups. Additionally, aphakic/pseudophakic eyes with a ruptured posterior capsule had a lower cure rate than phakic eyes, regardless of the technique used. Morbidity was less in the pneumatic retinopexy group. No cases of diplopia were reported, and minimal refractive changes were noted. Patients were rehabilitated faster because most individuals were not hospitalized, instead convalescing at home, and useful vision returned faster in this group. Pain, nausea, and proptosis were more severe and lasted longer in the scleral buckling group. At the 6-month postoperative period, 68% of eyes in the scleral buckle group were at least 1 D more myopic than preoperatively, as opposed to 3% of pneumatic retinopexy eyes.[164]

Comparing the two groups,[149] progressive cataract development was noted in 47% of eyes after scleral buckling, in contrast to 19% of phakic eyes after pneumatic retinopexy. Cataract surgery was performed 4 times more frequently (18% versus 4%) in the scleral buckling group, yet a visually limiting cataract was not present in these eyes before detachment surgery.

Intraoperative or postoperative complications that could accelerate cataract formation could not be demonstrated in any eye that underwent cataract surgery during the 24-month follow-up period. Some investigators have postulated that relative anterior segment ischemia produced by an existing scleral buckle may be responsible for cataract formation.[149]

When comparing the significance of reoperations on visual recovery, the investigators[164] noted that the best visual acuities were obtained in eyes successfully reattached after initial pneumatic retinopexy. Failure of an initial pneumatic retinopexy did not subsequently adversely affect the eye's anatomy or visual recovery.

The poorest visual results occurred in eyes in which an initial scleral buckling procedure failed. The data demonstrate that initial pneumatic retinopexy does not adversely affect the final anatomic outcome even though the reattachment rate is higher in the scleral buckle group. Significantly, the final visual acuity was better in the pneumatic retinopexy group.[164]

Both the 6- and 24-month evaluations indicated that only one eye in each group developed a retinal detachment after 6 months. Vitreous incarceration in a needle site causing chronic traction after pneumatic retinopexy has been suggested by some investigators as a factor in late retinal detachment. Despite the occasional occurrences of late retinal tear formation from vitreous incarceration in a sclerotomy site after vitrectomy, data show no difference in percentage of retinal detachments between the pneumatic retinopexy and scleral buckle groups.

Pneumatic retinopexy requires that the surgeon identify all retinal breaks before surgery and properly position the patient for 16 hours a day over a 5-day period; this requirement may be too difficult for some patients.[149] Pneumatic retinopexy is less expensive than scleral buckling, which may be significant to health care providers.[149] New breaks occurred more frequently in the pneumatic retinopexy group but did not adversely affect the outcome. Postoperative pain and pseudoptosis were more severe and lasted longer in the scleral buckling group.[164]

Myopic refractive shifts occurred in 3% of eyes in the pneumatic retinopexy and 68% in the scleral buckling group.[159,164]

MANAGEMENT OF SUBRETINAL AIR DURING AIR–FLUID EXCHANGE AFTER VITRECTOMY

Although it is a rare complication, air can gain access into subretinal space through existing retinal tears. Untreated, this condition can lead to failure of surgery and persistent retinal detachment.

Management of subretinal air involves creation of a sufficiently large anterior retinotomy through which gas or air can exit the subretinal space. To facilitate the exit of subretinal air, infusion fluid or perfluorocarbon liquid can be injected into the vitreous cavity to fill the cavity and force the subretinal gas through an existing retinotomy (Fig. 2–25). Rotating the eye to position the retinotomy in the superior aspect of the globe facilitates exit of the subretinal air through the retinotomy.

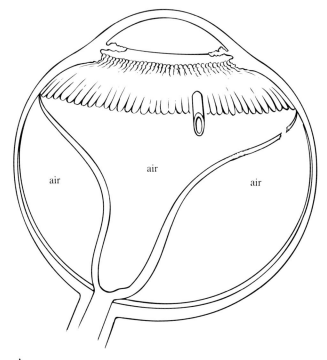

A

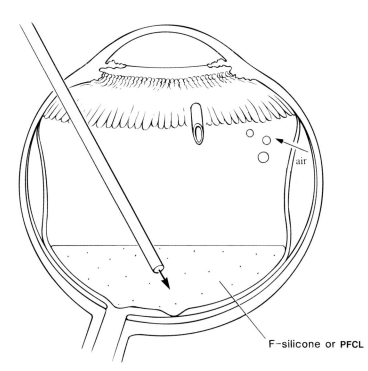

F-silicone or PFCL

B

OTHER USES OF AIR OR GAS IN VITREORETINAL SURGERY

Simultaneous External Drainage of Subretinal Fluid and Intravitreal Gas Injection

Meyers and FitzGibbon[182] developed a technique of simultaneous external subretinal fluid drainage and intravitreal gas injection.[182] This technique is useful in selected patients who have the form of retinal detachment often associated with PVR, who do not have a posterior retinal break to drain subretinal fluid, and who require a large or near total gas fill. After vitrectomy, a limited air–fluid exchange is performed, followed by closure of the two superior sclerotomies. The surgeon monitors the drainage of subretinal fluid through an external drainage site located 2 to 3 mm posterior to the equator and kept in a dependent position, when necessary, by rotating the eye. Simultaneously, intravitreal gas or air is injected into the eye. In vitrectomized eyes, a pressure-dependent air pump can be used for intravitreal air injection.

Simultaneous Perfusion of Air and Irrigating Solution in the Management of Traumatic Posterior Segment Injuries

Penetrating posterior segment injuries associated with posterior retinal perforation, retinal detachment, and vitreous hemorrhage are difficult to manage. During vitrectomy, infusion fluid can flow through the retinal tear, leading to further separation of the retina and the production of a bullous detachment (Fig 2–26A, B). A bullously detached retina can then become caught in the vitrectomy instrument, producing iatrogenic holes. We use a technique that simplifies the management of posterior retinal injuries (tears) associated with retinal detachments.[183]

A conjunctival peritomy is performed, and three sclerotomies are made at the pars plicata. One sclerotomy is for the full-function vitrectomy instrument (irrigation, aspiration, and cutting), one for a fiberoptic probe, and the third for an infusion cannula. Because lens damage commonly occurs with severe penetrating injuries of the posterior segment, a lensectomy and a limited anterior vitrectomy are done with the vitrectomy instrument (an ultrasonic unit may be used to remove a hard lens). At this time, the infusion cannula is switched to an air pump system, which provides a constant flow of air.[184] The air pressure is adjusted to 40 to 50 mm Hg. Usually the anterior chamber and anterior part of the vitreous cavity fill with air as the fluid escapes through the pars plana sclerotomies. Then a full-function vitrectomy instrument (V-19 Vitrophage, Vitrophage, Inc., Lyons, IL) is inserted inside the eye to provide infusion fluid. As long as the amount of irrigation fluid equals the amount being aspirated through the vitrectomy instrument, the air compartment inside the eye remains unchanged in size. After opacities in the anterior vitreous are removed, more

Figure 2–25. Management of subretinal air. **A.** Graphic representation of air under the retina. **B.** A peripheral retinotomy is performed, and PFCL is injected into the eye, forcing air through the peripheral retinotomy.

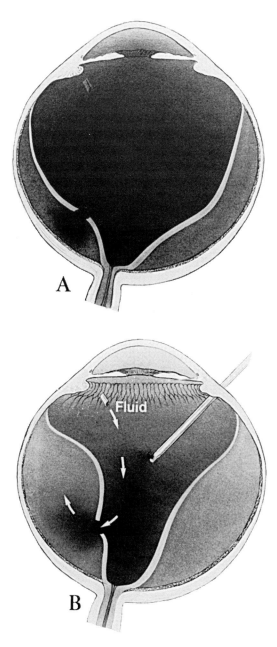

Figure 2–26. A. Artist's representation of a traumatic eye injury with vitreous hemorrhage and retinal detachment. **B.** The vitrectomy infusion fluid flows through the retinal tear, producing a bullous detachment.

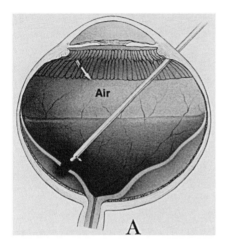

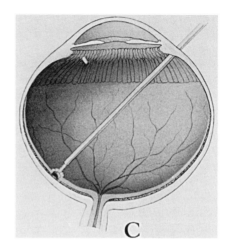

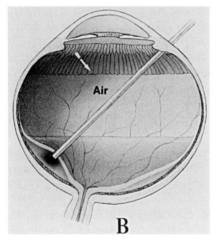

Figure 2–27. A. Artist's representation of how the air-filled compartment keeps the peripheral retina attached, while irrigation and aspiration are performed beneath the air-filled cavity. **B.** Subretinal fluid is drained, and the vitreous cavity is completely filled with air. **C.** Endolaser coagulation is applied to the retinal and choroidal wound.

liquid vitreous is aspirated than is being irrigated, to allow the anterior air-filled compartment to expand toward the posterior vitreous (Fig. 2–27A). Any remaining vitreous opacities are removed gradually by cutting and using lavage beneath the air-filled anterior vitreous cavity.

Because the air in the anterior chamber neutralizes the refractive power of the cornea, no contact lens is needed to visualize the posterior pole through the operating microscope. Furthermore, the air pressure in the anterior part of the vitreous pushes and holds the peripheral retina against the pigment epithelium, preventing its detachment (Fig. 2–27A). As the air compartment expands, the more peripheral portion of the retina can reattach. Finally, subretinal fluid is drained through an existing posterior retinal tear (Fig. 2–27B), and blood is cleared from the vitreous cavity and replaced with infusion fluid and air.

If there is an active choroidal hemorrhage, this technique contains the blood in the posterior, fluid-filled compartment, where it can be washed out and aspirated without disturbing the surgeon's view, using the full-function vitrectomy instrument. At the end of the procedure, the entire vitreous cavity is filled with air, and the retinal and choroidal injury sites are coagulated with the use of an endolaser (Fig. 2–27C). The air pump not only keeps the IOP under precise control, but it also aids in visualization of the fundus.

One advantage of this technique is the creation of an opacity-free medium in the anterior chamber and in the anterior vitreous cavity. Even if bleeding occurs in the posterior segment, the air bubble keeps the anterior part of the eye clear for undisturbed visualization. In addition, the danger of producing a bullously detached retina is eliminated, because the peripheral part of the retina is compressed against the eye wall by the pressure of the air-filled compartment. The operator can increase or decrease this air compartment selectively by aspirating more vitreous fluid than is being infused for irrigation. To decrease the air compartment, more irrigation fluid is infused, while some of the air is aspirated.

A disadvantage of the technique is that fluid is forced posteriorly and may detach the macula. Therefore, this technique should only be used in cases in which the macula is already detached. Also, air can cause miosis, but visualization can be increased by performing a limited iridectomy.

Surgeons who do not have full-function vitrectomy instrumentation may modify the technique by using two infusion cannulas: one connected to air, the other to infusion fluid.

THE USE OF AIR AND GAS IN THE TREATMENT OF GIANT RETINAL TEAR

Giant retinal breaks have been defined as those that extend 90° or more over the circumference of the fundus.[185] Management of retinal detachments resulting from giant retinal breaks remains one of the most difficult challenges in vitreoretinal surgery, especially when the breaks are associated with inversion of the posterior

Figure 2–28. Schematic drawing demonstrating management of giant retinal tear. **A.** Complete vitrectomy using vitrectomy instrument and endoilluminator. **B.** Pre-placement of buckle (posterior to equator) and injection of a small air bubble in the eye before rotation. **C** (page 116). Beginning rotation of the patient. Note that the tear passes initially through the most dependent (inferior) position. **D** (page 116). Complete air–fluid exchange using a needle and cannula. **E** (page 117). Completion of the patient's rotation. Air is constantly infused through the cannula. **F** (page 117). Tightening of the buckle and performing penetrating diathermy. **G** (page 118). Magnified view of the penetrating diathermy area. **H** (page 118). Demonstrating the diathermy effect, escape of air through the micropuncture after removal of the needle, and production of retinal microincarceration. **I** (page 118). Completion of the procedure. Cryotherapy is applied anterior to the buckle.

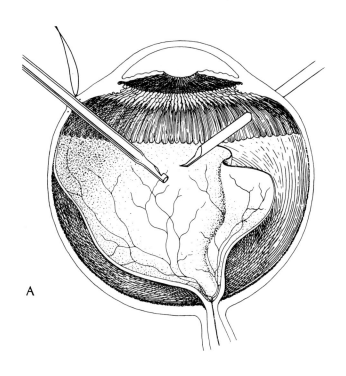

A

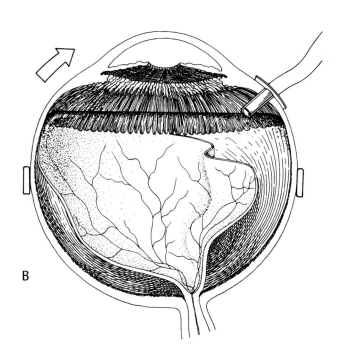

B

115

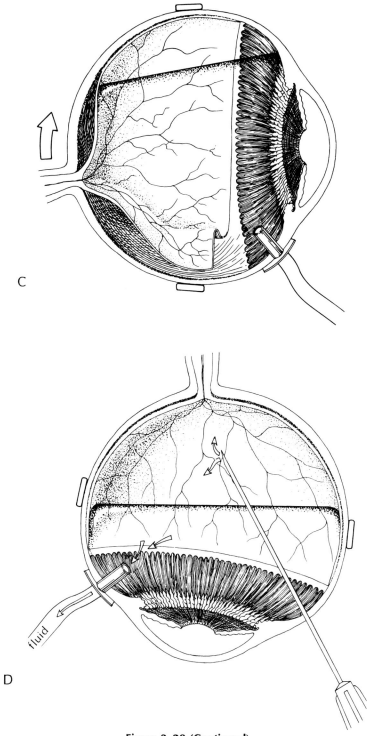

C

D

fluid

Figure 2–28 (Continued).

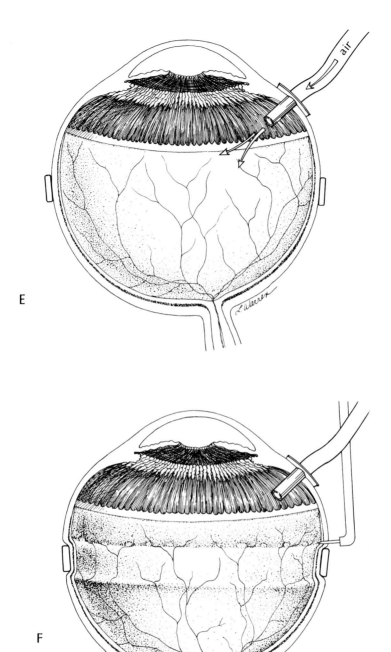

E

F

Figure 2–28 (Continued).

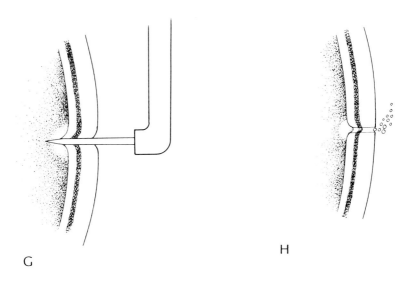

G

H

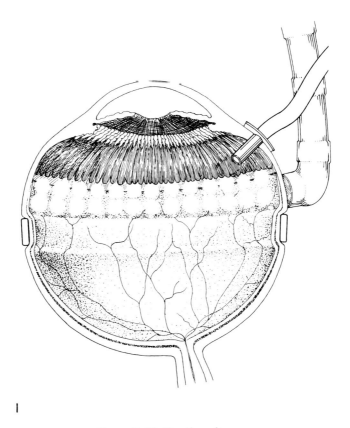

I

Figure 2–28 (Continued).

retinal flap. The overall success of these cases depends on intraoperative repositioning and fixation of the retina and postoperative measures to combat redetachment.

Generally, giant retinal tears respond poorly to conventional scleral buckling techniques,[186] even though a simple giant tear may be repaired with scleral buckling.[187,188] The prognosis for patients with giant retinal tears improved with the advent of vitrectomy,[189] a surgical procedure that allows direct release of traction on the retinal flap and allows the vitreous cavity to be filled with tamponading agents.[186,189]

In the past, techniques to reposition the retina by placing the patient in a supine position were rarely successful.[190-192] Vitrectomy, however, relieves the traction on the posterior retinal flap and allows complete fluid–air exchange[9,189] when used with a rotating table (Fig. 2–28).[193,194] The retina can then be repositioned more easily.

To maintain the retina in the proper place, an encircling band and intraocular SF_6 or C_3F_8 were used to tamponade[189] the repositioned retina while either surface diathermy[194] or cryocoagulation[195] achieved chorioretinal adhesion. However, both diathermy and cryocoagulation encourage subretinal exudate formation, and it is possible for the posterior flap of the tear to slide further posteriorly after surgery. This may allow the retina to float free before adhesion becomes permanent. To fix the repositioned retina, some surgeons advocated incarceration of the retina in a sclerotomy by forcing drainage of subretinal fluid.[196] Other surgeons employed drainage of vitreous anterior to the tear to reposition and flatten the retina.[197] These techniques, however, were complicated by retinal folds, at times creating tracks in the eye for infection or fibrous ingrowth.

Other methods of retinal fixation have included transscleral suturing[198-200] and open-sky transvitreal retinal suturing alone[201] or in conjunction with subtotal open-sky vitrectomy.[202,203] Both techniques are difficult, time consuming, and can cause vitreous and choroidal hemorrhage.[202]

A technique described by Peyman and co-workers[196] simplified retinal fixation by producing microincarceration of the retina with a sharp penetrating diathermy needle. After retinal reattachment and air–fluid exchange, the diathermy needle penetrated the sclera. The choroid and retina were melted together by the coagulative action of the diathermy. In addition, removal of the needle forced the air into the needle tract, producing microincarceration.

Surgical techniques have been used to reposition and fix the inverted retinal flap with the patient remaining supine during the entire procedure. These techniques include intravitreal injection of perfluorocarbon gases without vitrectomy[204] or drainage; the use of Healon[192,205] (Kabi Pharmacia Ophthalmics, Menrovia, CA) or fluorosilicone[206] to unfold a giant tear; and postoperative repositioning of the patient to reattach the retina.[207,208]

Other procedures have been described that use vitrectomy combined with silicone oil[186,209] or gas.[186,210] A cannulated extrusion needle has also been used in conjunction with vitrectomy and fluid–gas exchange to drain subretinal fluid and reposition the tear.[210] The additional use of delamination, membrane peeling, or segmentation has successfully relieved retinal traction in many instances of giant retinal tear.[211]

OTHER METHODS OF USING AIR IN THE MANAGEMENT OF GIANT RETINAL TEAR

Glaser[210,212] described a technique involving fluid–gas exchange with the patient kept in a supine position to treat giant retinal tears complicated by proliferative vitreoretinopathy. A vitrectomy is performed. The lens is removed in phakic eyes, and an inferior iridectomy is performed with the vitrectomy probe.

An air–fluid exchange is initiated, filling the anterior chamber with air. A soft-tipped 20-gauge flute needle with reflux capabilities is introduced into the eye, and the tip is placed just above the most anterior part of the torn retina. Using an air pump, the fluid–gas exchange is continued until the bubble extends to the edge of the retina. After removal of all fluid from this area, the air bubble traps the retina against the RPE.

Joondeph and associates[213] described the management of giant retinal tears with the cannulated extrusion needle. After vitrectomy with removal of all preretinal membranes and any vitreous adherent to the posterior edge of the tear, transvitreal diathermy is used to mark the posterior edge of the tear, facilitating later identification in the air-filled eye.

The giant tear is placed in the most dependent position by rotating the eye or turning the head. Using the light pipe and cannulated extrusion needle, the tear is unfolded and manipulated as far anterior as possible. A continuous air–fluid exchange is performed. The cannulated extrusion needle is passed posteriorly through the giant tear to remove subretinal fluid while the air meniscus descends to the level of the giant tear. The retina should be flat when the eye is completely filled with air.

Williams et al,[214] using a two-stage technique for intraoperative fluid–gas exchange after vitrectomy, reported intraoperative reattachment of all 18 eyes with a mean follow-up of 11 months, but eight eyes redetached during this period, requiring additional surgery.

Repair of Giant Retinal Tears Without Scleral Buckling

Giant retinal tears with complicated retinal detachments involving PVR often require the use of peripheral encircling elements; however, the repair of giant retinal tears can be performed without the use of scleral buckling. Hoffman and Sorr[208] described the repair of giant retinal tears with preoperative panretinal photocoagulation to peripherally attached retina followed by pars plana vitrectomy, transscleral cryopexy, and injection of a bubble of pure C_3F_8. Postoperative positioning promoted flattening of the retina in all patients. They concluded that scleral buckling may not be needed in the absence of retinal foreshortening and transretinal traction. Other complications, such as anterior redundant retinal folds, posterior radial folds, fish-mouthing of the retinal break, and choroidal detachments, may be avoided when the scleral buckle is not used in the repair of giant retinal tears.[208]

USE OF INTRAVITREAL GAS AFTER FAILURE OF SCLERAL BUCKLING PROCEDURES

Retinal detachment surgery fails in 5% to 10% of eyes. Morbidity, the development of PVR, and the risk of complications are increased by surgical revision.

Worsley and Grey[215] used four criteria for the use of supplemental intravitreal gas after failure of scleral buckling procedures in eyes with rhegmatogenous retinal detachment. An open break had to be visible between the 8 o'clock and 4 o'clock positions in the presence of a documented increase or reappearance of subretinal fluid. Additionally, the open retinal tears had to be in the correct position in relationship to an underlying scleral buckle of adequate height. Injection of 0.5 to 0.8 mL 100% SF_6 was performed in 11 eyes; seven eyes met the four criteria, and the other four were judged likely to benefit from the procedure despite the inadequacy of the buckle. Gas was removed if closure of the central retinal artery was observed. The patients were positioned so as to achieve gas tamponade of the retinal breaks; positioning was maintained for 2 to 5 days. When retinal reapposition was achieved, the sufficiency of cryotherapy surrounding the break was evaluated. If the cryotherapy was judged to be inadequate or if it had been applied more than 7 days before, then laser photocoagulation spots were placed around the retinal breaks. Successful retinal reattachment was achieved in all seven eyes meeting selection criteria; the other four eyes were anatomic failures. PVR occurred in two of the four patients with unsuccessful retinal reattachment; no complications were observed in the eyes with anatomically successful reattachment. Follow-up ranged from 3 to 12 months.[215]

USE OF AIR AS A HEMOSTATIC AGENT

Joondeph and Blankenship[213] evaluated the hemostatic effects of an intravitreal air bubble in experimental animal vitrectomy and in diabetic patients undergoing vitrectomy. Previously, the tamponading effect of intraocular air or gas on bleeding sites was believed to allow hemostasis to occur through natural clotting mechanisms, thereby preventing postoperative hemorrhage. These two studies indicated that intravitreal air does not improve hemostasis perioperatively or after diabetic vitrectomy, but does probably increase the incidence of cataract formation.[213,216]

REFERENCES

1. Ohm J: Über die Behandlung der Netzhautablösung durch operative Entleerung der Subretinalen Flüssigkeit und Einspritzung von Luft in den Glaskörper. *Albrecht von Graefes Arch Ophthalmol* 1911;79:442–465.
2. Rosengren B: Über die Behandlung der Netzhautablösung mittelst Diathermie und Luftinjektion in den Glaskörper. *Acta Ophthalmol* 1938;16:3–42.

3. Rosengren B: Air injection in retinal detachment, in *XVI Concilium Ophthalmologicum Britannia, 1950, ACTA*. London: British Medical Association, 1951, pp 1212–1217.

4. Rosengren B: 300 cases operated upon for retinal detachment: Method and results. *Acta Ophthalmol* 1952;30:117–122.

5. Chawla HB: Intravitreal air in aphakic retinal detachment. *Br J Ophthalmol* 1973; 57:58–59.

6. Chawla HB, Birchall CH: Intravitreal air in retinal detachment surgery. *Br J Ophthalmol* 1973;57:60–70.

7. Arruga H: Certain considerations of the surgical treatment of retinal detachment. *Am J Ophthalmol* 1952;35:1573–1580.

8. Pillat A: Ergebnisse mit der Luftinjektion in den Glaskorper nach diathermischer Operation gegen Netzhautablosung. *Ver Oster Ophthalmol Ges* 1957;3:57.

9. Norton EWD, Aaberg T, Fung W, et al: Giant retinal tears: I. Clinical management with intravitreal air. *Am J Ophthalmol* 1969;68:1011–1021.

10. Machemer R, Aaberg TM, Norton EWD: Giant retinal tears: II. Experimental production and management with intravitreal air. *Am J Ophthalmol* 1969; 68:1022–1029.

11. Schenk H: Experimentelle und klinische Untersuchungen zur Frage der Resorption gasförmiger Stoffe aus dem Glaskörper. *Albrecht von Graefes Arch Ophthalmol* 1959;161:252–281.

12. Widder W: Tierversuche über die Verweildauer verschiedener Glaskörperimplantate. *Albrecht von Graefes Arch Ophthalmol* 1962;164:550–569.

13. Vygantas CM, Peyman GA, Daily MJ, et al: Octafluorocyclobutane and other gases for vitreous replacement. *Arch Ophthalmol* 1973;90:235–236.

14. Tanenbaum HL: Gas injection in the rabbit vitreous: A preliminary study. *Can J Ophthalmol* 1972;7:349–351.

15. Crittenden JJ, de Juan E, Tiedeman J: Expansion of long-acting gas bubbles for intraocular use: Principles and practices. *Arch Ophthalmol* 1985;103:831–834.

16. Piiper J, Canfield RE, Rahn H: Absorption of various inert gases from subcutaneous gas pockets in rats. *J Appl Physiol* 1962;17:268–274.

17. Tucker RW, Tenney SM: Inert gas exchange in subcutaneous gas pockets of air-breathing animals: Theory and measurement. *Respir Physiol* 1966;1:151–171.

18. Tenney SM, Carpenter FG, Rahn H: Gas transfers in a sulfur hexafluoride pneumoperitoneum. *J Appl Physiol* 1953;6:201–208.

19. Peters MA, Abrams GW, Hamilton LH, et al: The nonexpansile, equilibrated concentration of perfluoropropane gas in the eye. *Am J Ophthalmol* 1985; 100:831–839.

20. Abrams GW, Edelhauser HF, Aaberg TM, et al: Dynamics of intravitreal sulfur hexafluoride gas. *Invest Ophthalmol* 1974;13:863–868.

21. Sendroy J Jr, Collison HA: Solubility of SF_6 in biologic fluids. *Fed Proc* 1955;14:279.

22. Lopez R, Chang S: Long-term results of vitrectomy and perfluorocarbon gas for the treatment of severe proliferative vitreoretinopathy. *Am J Ophthalmol* 1992;113:424–428.

23. Killey FP, Edelhauser HF, Aaberg TM: Intraocular sulfur hexafluoride and octafluorocyclobutane: Effects on intraocular pressure and vitreous volume. *Arch Ophthalmol* 1978;96:511–515.

24. Lincoff H, Ramirez V, Mohr D: An investigation of gases for intravitreal injection. Read before the Cornell Eye Alumni Meeting, New York, 1968.

25. Norton EWD: Intraocular gas in the management of selected retinal detachments. *Trans Am Acad Ophthalmol Otolaryngol* 1973;77:OP85–OP98.

26. Aaberg TM, Abrams GW, Edelhauser HF: Intraocular sulfur hexafluoride: An experimental and clinical correlation, in McPherson A (ed): *New and Controversial Aspects of Vitreoretinal Surgery.* St Louis: CV Mosby, 1977, pp 393–396.

27. Fineberg E, Machemer R, Sullivan P, et al: Sulfur hexafluoride in owl monkey vitreous cavity. *Am J Ophthalmol* 1975;79:67–76.

28. Van Horn DL, Edelhauser HF, Aaberg TM, et al: In vivo effects of air and sulfur hexafluoride gas on rabbit corneal endothelium. *Invest Ophthalmol* 1972; 11:1028–1036.

29. Sabates WI, Abrams GW, Swanson DE, et al: The use of intraocular gases: The results of sulfur hexafluoride gas in retinal detachment surgery. *Ophthalmology* 1981;88:447–454.

30. Abrams GW, Swanson DE, Sabates WI: The results of sulfur hexafluoride gas in vitreous surgery. *Am J Ophthalmol* 1982;94:165–171.

31. Taylor GJ IV, Harris WS, Bogdonoff MD: Ventricular arrhythmias induced in monkeys by the inhalation of aerosol propellants. *J Clin Invest* 1971;50:1546–1550.

32. Brubaker S, Peyman GA, Vygantas, C: Toxicity of octafluorocyclobutane after intracameral injection. *Arch Ophthalmol* 1974;92:324–328.

33. Peyman GA, Vygantas CM, Bennett TO, et al: Octafluorocyclobutane in vitreous and aqueous humor replacement. *Arch Ophthalmol* 1975;93:514–517.

34. Lincoff A, Haft D, Liggett P, et al: Intravitreal expansion of perfluorocarbon bubbles. *Arch Ophthalmol* 1980;98:1646.

35. Bochow TW, Olk RJ, Hershey JM: Pneumatic retinopexy perfluoroethane (C_2F_6) in the treatment of rhegmatogenous retinal detachment. *Arch Ophthalmol* 1992; 110:1723–1724.

36. Lincoff H, Coleman J, Kressig I, et al: The perfluorocarbon gases in the treatment of retinal detachment. *Ophthalmology* 1983;90:546–551.

37. Peyman GA, Namperumalsamy P, Vygantas C: Clinical trial of intravitreal C_4F_8 in retinal detachment surgery. *Can J Ophthalmol* 1975;10:218–221.

38. Lincoff A, Lincoff H, Iwamoto T, et al: Perfluoro-n-butane: A gas for a maximum duration retinal tamponade. *Arch Ophthalmol* 1983;101:460–462.

39. Wong RF, Thompson JT: The prediction of the kinetics of disappearance of sulfur hexafluoride and perfluoropropane intraocular gas bubbles. *Ophthalmology* 1988; 95:609–613.

40. Lincoff H, Mardirossian J, Lincoff A, et al: Intravitreal longevity of three perfluorocarbon gases. *Arch Ophthalmol* 1980;98:1610–1611.

41. Chang S: Intraocular gases, in Ryan SJ (ed): *Retina,* vol. 3. St. Louis; CV Mosby, 1989, pp 245–259.

42. Meyers SM, Ambler JS, Tan M, et al: Variation of perfluoropropane disappearance after vitrectomy. *Retina* 1992;12:359–363.

43. Jacobs P: Estimating intraocular gas volume. *Ophthalmology* 1988;95:1481.

44. Jacobs PM, Twomey JM, Leaver PK: Behaviour of intraocular gases. *Eye* 1988; 2:660–663.

45. Thompson JT: Kinetics of intraocular gases: Disappearance of air, sulfur hexafluoride, and perfluoropropane after pars plana vitrectomy. *Arch Ophthalmol* 1989;107:687–691.

46. Thompson JT: The absorption of mixtures of air and perfluoropropane after pars plana vitrectomy. *Arch Ophthalmol* 1992;110:1594–1597.

47. Lincoff H, Maisel JM, Lincoff A: Intravitreal disappearance rates of four perfluorocarbon gases. *Arch Ophthalmol* 1984;102:928–929.

48. Yanoff M: Anatomy of the human eye, in Scheie HG, Albert DM (eds): *Textbook of Ophthalmology*, ed 4. Philadelphia: WB Saunders, 1977, pp 45–78.

49. Prince JH, McConnell DG: Retina and optic nerve, in Prince JH (ed): *The Rabbit in Eye Research*. Springfield, IL: Charles C Thomas, 1964, p 388.

50. Lincoff H, Stergiu P, Smith R, et al: Longevity of expanding gas in vitrectomized eyes. *Retina* 1992;12:364–366.

51. Fisher YL, Shakin JL, Slakter JS, et al: Perfluoropropane gas, modified panretinal photocoagulation, and vitrectomy in the management of severe proliferative vitreoretinopathy. *Arch Ophthalmol* 1988;106:1255–1260.

52. Brinton DA, Hilton GF: Pneumatic retinopexy. *Ophthalmology Clin North Am* 1994;7:1–12.

53. Gardner TW, Norris JL, Zakov ZN, et al: A survey of intraocular gas use in North America. *Arch Ophthalmol* 1988;106:1188–1189.

54. Ai E, Gardner TW: Current patterns of intraocular gas use in North America. *Arch Ophthalmol* 1993;111:331–332.

55. Parver LM, Lincoff H: Geometry of intraocular gas used in retinal surgery. *Mod Probl Ophthalmol* 1977;18:338–343.

56. Parver LM, Lincoff H: Mechanics of intraocular gas. *Invest Ophthalmol Vis Sci* 1978;17:77–79.

57. Jacobs PM: Intraocular gas measurement using A-scan ultrasound. *Curr Eye Res* 1986;5:575–578.

58. Foulks GN, de Juan E, Hatchell DL, et al: The effect of perfluoropropane on the cornea in rabbits and cats. *Arch Ophthalmol* 1987;105:256–259.

59. Lee DA, Wilson R, Yoshizumi MO, et al: The ocular effects of gases when injected into the anterior chamber of rabbit eyes. *Arch Ophthalmol* 1991;109:571–575.

60. Lincoff H, Kreissig I: Posterior lip traction caused by intravitreal gas. *Arch Ophthalmol* 1981;99:1367–1370.

61. Ogura Y, Tsukada T, Negi A, et al: Integrity of the blood–ocular barrier after intravitreal gas injection. *Retina* 1989;9:199–202.

62. Sparrow JR, Chang S, Gershbein A, et al: MRI studies of blood–ocular barriers with intravitreal gas. *Invest Ophthalmol Vis Sci* 1990;31(Suppl):23.

63. Wong RF, Liggett PE: Intraocular inflammation following intravitreal gas injection. *Invest Ophthalmol Vis Sci* 1990;31(suppl):438.

64. Lincoff H, Kreissig I: Application of xenon gas to clinical retinal detachment. *Arch Ophthalmol* 1982;100:1083–1085.

65. Lincoff A, Lincoff H, Solorzano C, et al: Selection of xenon gas for rapidly disappearing retinal tamponade. *Arch Ophthalmol* 1982;100:996–997.

66. Wolf GL, Capuano C, Hartung J: Effect of nitrous oxide on gas bubble volume in the anterior chamber. *Arch Ophthalmol* 1985;103:418–419.

67. Michels RG: Scleral buckling methods for rhegmatogenous retinal detachment. *Retina* 1986;6:1–49.

68. Munson ES, Eger EI II, Tham MK, et al: Increase in anesthetic uptake, excretion, and blood solubility in man after eating. *Anesth Analg* 1978;57:224–231.

69. Eger EI: *Nitrous Oxide, N_2O*. New York: Elsevier Science, 1985, pp 100–102.

70. Stinson TW III, Donlon JV Jr: Interaction of intraocular air and sulfur hexafluoride with nitrous oxide: A computer simulation. *Anesthesiology* 1982;56:385–388.
71. Smith RB, Carl B, Linn JG, et al: Effect of nitrous oxide on air in vitreous. *Am J Ophthalmol* 1974;78:314–317.
72. Aronowitz JD, Brubaker RF: Effect of intraocular gas on intraocular pressure. *Arch Ophthalmol* 1976;94:1191–1196.
73. Schwartz A: Chronic open-angle glaucoma secondary to rhegmatogenous retinal detachment. *Trans Am Ophthalmol Soc* 1972;70:178–189.
74. Matsuo N, Takabatake M, Ueno H, et al: Photoreceptor outer segments in the aqueous humor in rhegmatogenous retinal detachment. *Am J Ophthalmol* 1986; 101:673–679.
75. Simone JN, Whitacre MM: The effect of intraocular gas and fluid volumes on intraocular pressure. *Ophthalmology* 1990;97:238–243.
76. Smith TR: Acute glaucoma developing after scleral buckling procedures. *Am J Ophthalmol* 1967;63:1807–1808.
77. Frenkel REP, Hong YJ, Shin DH: Comparison of the Tono-Pen to the Goldmann applanation tonometer. *Arch Ophthalmol* 1988;106:750–753.
78. Moses RA: Schiotz tonometry with an air bubble in the eye. *Am J Ophthalmol* 1966;62:281–282.
79. Kaufman HE: Pressure measurement: Which tonometer? *Invest Ophthalmol* 1972; 11:80–85.
80. McMillan F, Forster RK: Comparison of MacKay-Marg, Goldmann and Perkins tonometers in abnormal corneas. *Arch Ophthalmol* 1975;93:420–424.
81. Kaufman HE, West CE, Wood TO, et al: Measurement and control of intraocular pressure in corneal disease. *Int Ophthalmol Clin* 1970;10:387–401.
82. Wind CA, Irvine AR: Electronic applanation tonometry in corneal edema and keratoplasty. *Invest Ophthalmol* 1969;8:620–624.
83. Rootman DS, Insler MS, Thompson HW, et al: Accuracy and precision of the Tono-Pen in measuring intraocular pressure after keratoplasty and epikeratophakia and in scarred corneas. *Arch Ophthalmol* 1988;106:1697–1700.
84. Hessemer V, Rössler R, Jacobi KW: Comparison of intraocular pressure measurements with the Oculab Tono-Pen vs manometry in humans shortly after death. *Am J Ophthalmol* 1988;105:678–682.
85. Mendelsohn AD, Forster RK, Mendelsohn SL, et al: Comparative tonometric measurements of eye bank eyes. *Cornea* 1987;6:219–225.
86. Boothe WA, Lee DA, Panek WC, et al: The Tono-Pen: A manometric and clinical study. *Arch Ophthalmol* 1988;106:1214–1217.
87. Armstrong TA: Evaluation of the Tono-Pen and the Pulsar tonometers. *Am J Ophthalmol* 1990;109:716–720.
88. Hines MW, Jost BF, Fogelman KL: Oculab Tono-Pen, Goldmann applanation tonometry, and pneumatic tonometry for intraocular pressure assessment in gas-filled eyes. *Am J Ophthalmol* 1988;106:174–179.
89. Minckler DS, Baerveldt G, Heuer DK, et al: Clinical evaluation of the Oculab Tono-Pen. *Am J Ophthalmol* 1987;104:168–173.
90. Anderson DR, Grant WM: The influence of position on intraocular pressure. *Invest Ophthalmol* 1973;12:204–212.
91. Del Priore LV, Michels RG, Nunez MA, et al: Intraocular pressure measurement after pars plana vitrectomy. *Ophthalmology* 1989;96:1353–1356.
92. Badrinath SG, Ramabudhra V, Murugesan R, et al: Intraoperative measurement of

intraocular pressure in vitrectomized aphakic air-filled eyes using the Tono-Pen SL. *Retina* 1993;13:307–311.

93. Lim JI, Blair NP, Higginbotham EJ, et al: Assessment of intraocular pressure in vitrectomized gas-containing eyes: A clinical and manometric comparison of the Tono-Pen to the pneumotonometer. *Arch Ophthalmol* 1990;108:684–688.

94. Landers MB III, Robinson D, Olsen KR, et al: Slit-lamp fluid-gas exchange and other office procedures following vitreoretinal surgery. *Arch Ophthalmol* 1985; 103:967–972.

95. Lincoff H, Kreissig I, Brodie S, et al: Expanding gas bubbles for the repair of tears in the posterior pole. *Graefes Arch Clin Exp Ophthalmol* 1982;219:193–197.

96. Bloch D, O'Conner P, Lincoff H: The mechanism of the cryosurgical adhesion: III. Statistical analysis. *Am J Ophthalmol* 1971;71:666–673.

97. Han DP, Abrams GW, Bennett SR, et al: Perfluoropropane 12% versus 20%: Effect on intraocular pressure and gas tamponade after pars plana vitrectomy. *Retina* 1993;13:302–306.

98. Twomey JM, Leaver PK: Retinal compression folds. *Eye* 1988;2:273–287.

99. Lewen RM, Lyon CE, Diamond JG: Scleral buckling with intraocular air injection complicated by arcuate retinal folds. *Arch Ophthalmol* 1987;105:1212–1214.

100. Larrison WI, Fredrick AR Jr, Paterson TJ, et al: Posterior retinal folds following vitreoretinal surgery. *Arch Ophthalmol* 1993;111:621–625.

101. Humayun MS, Yeo JH, Koski WS, et al: The rate of sulfur hexafluoride escape from a plastic syringe. *Arch Ophthalmol* 1989;107:853–854.

102. Cummings HL, Haller J, Koski WS: Perfluoropropane and sulfur hexafluoride: Diffusion rates from a plastic syringe and accuracy of volume based gas air mixing. *Invest Ophthalmol Vis Sci* 1990;31(Suppl):23.

103. Raymond G, Jasicniak M, Wong HC: Long-term storage of perfluoropropane (C_3F_8) in plastic syringes. *Retina* 1993;13:80–81.

104. Friedrichsen EJ, McMullen WW, Garcia CA: Storage of sulfur hexafluoride gas. *Ophthalmic Surg* 1993;24:62.

105. Friedrichsen EJ, McMullen WW, Garcia CA: Sulfahexafluoride gas delivery, storage, and mass analysis using Vacutainer (TM) tubes: An analysis of percentage delivery, gas chromatography and serial measurements to evaluate tube leakage. *Invest Ophthalmol Vis Sci* 1992;33(Suppl):1315.

106. De Juan E Jr, McCuen B, Tiedeman J: Intraocular tamponade and surface tension. *Surv Ophthalmol* 1985;30:47–51.

107. Stern WH, Johnson RN, Irvine AR, et al: Extended retinal tamponade in the treatment of retinal detachment with proliferative vitreoretinopathy. *Br J Ophthalmol* 1986;70:911–917.

108. Yeo JH, Michels RG: Preoperative laser photocoagulation to mark tiny retinal breaks in eyes with retinal detachment. *Retina* 1985;5:161–162.

109. Fisher YL, Sorenson JA: Retinal tear localization following fluid–gas exchange during pars plana vitreoretinal surgery. *Am J Ophthalmol* 1984;97:390.

110. Peyman GA: An illuminated air–fluid switch for vitrectomy. *Retina* 1988;8:288.

111. Charles S: Fluid–gas exchange in the vitreous cavity. *Outcome Newsletter* 1977;2:1–2.

112. Peyman GA, Sanders DR: *Advances in Uveal Surgery, Vitreous Surgery, and the Treatment of Endophthalmitis.* New York: Appleton-Century-Crofts, 1975, pp 117–120.

113. Peyman GA: An illuminated suction needle for air–fluid exchange after vitrectomy. *Arch Ophthalmol* 1985;103:595–596.
114. Flynn HW, Lee WG, Parel J-M: Design features and surgical use of a cannulated extrusion needle. *Graefes Arch Clin Exp Ophthalmol* 1989;227:304–308.
115. Doft BH: Intentional retinotomy for internal drainage of subretinal fluid. *Arch Ophthalmol* 1986;104:807–808.
116. Živojnović R, Vijfuinkel G: A brush back-flush needle. *Arch Ophthalmol* 1988; 106:695.
117. Diddie KR, Smith RE: Intraocular gas injection in the pseudophakic patient. *Am J Ophthalmol* 1980;89:659–661.
118. Gonvers M: Retinal perforator for internal drainage. *Am J Ophthalmol* 1984; 97:786–787.
119. Fleishman J, Lerner BC, Reimels H: A new intraocular aspiration probe with bipolar cautery and reflux capabilities. *Arch Ophthalmol* 1989;107:283.
120. Davidorf FH, Chambers RB, Reimels HG: Evacuation/cautery vitreous needle. *Arch Ophthalmol* 1989;107:607.
121. Abrams GW: Retinotomies and retinectomies, vol. 3, in Ryan S (ed): *Retina*. St. Louis: CV Mosby, 1989, pp 317–346.
122. McDonald HR, Lewis HL, Aaberg TM, et al: Complications of endodrainage retinotomies created during vitreous surgery for complicated retinal detachment. *Ophthalmology* 1989;96:358–363.
123. Flynn HW Jr, Blumenkranz MS, Parel JM, et al: Cannulated subretinal fluid aspirator for vitreoretinal microsurgery. *Am J Ophthalmol* 1987;103:106–108.
124. Flynn HW, Davis JL, Parel JM, et al: Applications of a cannulated extrusion needle during vitreoretinal microsurgery. *Retina* 1988;8:42–49.
125. Flynn HW Jr, Lee WG, Parel JM: A simple extrusion needle with flexible cannula tip for vitreoretinal microsurgery. *Am J Ophthalmol* 1988;105:215–216.
126. Peyman GA: Letter to the editor. *Retina* 1988;8:221.
127. Blumenkranz M, Gardner T, Blankenship G: Fluid–gas exchange and photocoagulation after vitrectomy: Indications, technique, and results. *Arch Ophthalmol* 1986;104:291–296.
128. Chang S, Lincoff HA, Coleman DJ, et al: Perfluorocarbon gases in vitreous surgery. *Ophthalmology* 1985;92:651–656.
129. Stern WH, Blumenkranz MS: Fluid–gas exchange after vitrectomy. *Am J Ophthalmol* 1983;96:400–402.
130. Miller JA, Chandra SR, Stevens TS: A modified technique for performing outpatient fluid–air exchange following vitrectomy surgery. *Am J Ophthalmol* 1986;101: 116–117.
131. Lambrou FH, Devenyi RG, Han DP: Fluid–gas exchange after vitrectomy using long-acting gases in an outpatient setting. *Arch Ophthalmol* 1988;106:1344.
132. Kleiner RC: A new device for performing fluid–gas exchanges. *Arch Ophthalmol* 1988;106:421–422.
133. Barondes MJ, Davis MD, Myers FL: Acute glaucoma following fluid–gas exchange in a phakic patient. *Am J Ophthalmol* 1989;108:738–740.
134. Fuller D: Flying and intraocular gas bubble. *Am J Ophthalmol* 1981;91:276–277.
135. Brinkley JR Jr: Flying after vitreous injection. *Am J Ophthalmol* 1980;90:580–581.
136. Dieckert JP, O'Connor PS, Schacklett DE, et al: Air travel and intraocular gas. *Ophthalmology* 1986;93:642–645.

137. Lincoff H, Weinberger D, Reppucci V, et al: Air travel with intraocular gas: I. Mechanisms for compensation. *Arch Ophthalmol* 1989;107:902–906.
138. Lincoff H, Weinberger D, Stergiu P: Air travel with intraocular gas: II. Clinical considerations. *Arch Ophthalmol* 1989;107:907–910.
139. Domínguez AA: Cirugia precoz y ambulatoria del desprendimiento de retina. *Arch Soc Esp Oftalmol* 1985;48:47–54.
140. Hilton GF, Grizzard WS: Pneumatic retinopexy: A two step outpatient operation without conjunctival incision. *Ophthalmology* 1986;93:626–641.
141. Boyd BF: What is the most important, fairly simple to perform, new surgical technique for the management of retinal detachment: How do patients benefit? What are the indications, results, and step-by-step technique? *Highlights Ophthalmol Letter* 1986;14(5):1–14.
142. Tornambe PE: Bilateral retinal detachment repaired with bilateral pneumatic retinopexy. *Arch Ophthalmol* 1987;105:1489.
143. Hilton GF, Kelly NE, Salzano TC, et al: Pneumatic retinopexy: A collaborative report of the first 100 cases. *Ophthalmology* 1987;94:307–314.
144. Kamp-Mortensen K, Sjolie AK: Retinal detachment treated by pneumatic retinopexy. *Acta Ophthalmol* 1988;66:187–198.
145. Algvere P, Hallnäs K, Palmqvist B-M: Success and complications of pneumatic retinopexy. *Am J Ophthalmol* 1988;106:400–404.
146. Tornambe PE, Hilton GF, Kelly NF, et al: Expanded indications for pneumatic retinopexy. *Ophthalmology* 1988;95:597–600.
147. Friberg TR, Fourman SB: Scleral buckling and ocular rigidity: Clinical ramifications. *Arch Ophthalmol* 1990;108:1622–1627.
148. Hilton GF, Kelly NE, Tornambe PE: Extension of retinal detachments as a complication of pneumatic retinopexy. *Arch Ophthalmol* 1987;105:168.
149. Tornambe PE: Pneumatic retinopexy. *Surv Ophthalmol* 1988;32:270–281.
150. Tornambe PE: Pneumatic retinopexy: Current status and future directions. *Int Ophthalmol Clin* 1992;32(2):61–80.
151. Gunnerson G, Byhr E, Leyon H: Pneumatic retinopexy. *Acta Ophthalmol* 1990;68(Suppl):125–128.
152. Parver L: Intraocular gas tamponades used in retinal surgery. *Ann Ophthalmol* 1979;11:109–111.
153. Pallan LA, Eller AW, Friberg TR: Pneumatic retinopexy: An overview. *Semin Ophthalmol* 1991;6:27–35.
154. Friberg TR, Eller AW: Pneumatic repair of primary and secondary retinal detachments using a binocular indirect ophthalmoscope laser delivery system. *Ophthalmology* 1988;95:187–193.
155. Friberg TR: Clinical experience with a binocular indirect ophthalmoscope laser delivery system. *Retina* 1987;7:28–31.
156. Chen JC, Robertson JE, Coonan P, et al: Results and complications of pneumatic retinopexy. *Ophthalmology* 1988;95:601–608.
157. McAllister IL, Meyers SM, Zegarra H, et al: Comparison of pneumatic retinopexy with alternative surgical techniques. *Ophthalmology* 1988;95:877–883.
158. Lowe MA, McDonald R, Campo RV, et al: Pneumatic retinopexy: Surgical results. *Arch Ophthalmol* 1988;106:1672–1676.
159. Hilton GF, Tornambe PE, Retinal Detachment Study Group: Pneumatic retinopexy: An analysis of intraoperative and postoperative complications. *Retina* 1991;11:285–294.

160. Dreyer RF: Sequential retinal tears attributed to intraocular gas. *Am J Ophthalmol* 1986;102:276–278.
161. Freeman WR, Lipson BK, Morgan CM, et al: New posteriorly located retinal breaks after pneumatic retinopexy. *Ophthalmology* 1988;95:14–18.
162. Poliner LS, Grand MG, Schoch LH, et al: New retinal detachment after pneumatic retinopexy. *Ophthalmology* 1987;94:315–318.
163. Runge PE, Wyhinny GJ: Macular hole secondary to pneumatic retinopexy. *Arch Ophthalmol* 1988;106:586–587.
164. Tornambe PE, Hilton GF, The Retinal Detachment Study Group: Pneumatic retinopexy: A multicenter randomized controlled clinical trial comparing pneumatic retinopexy with scleral buckling. *Ophthalmology* 1989;96:772–784.
165. Ambler JS, Meyers SM, Zegarra H, et al: Reoperations and visual results after failed pneumatic retinopexy. *Ophthalmology* 1990;97:786–790.
166. Norton EWD: Retinal detachment in aphakia. *Am J Ophthalmol* 1964;58: 111–124.
167. Smiddy WE, Flynn HW Jr, Nicholson DH, et al: Results and complications in treated retinal breaks. *Am J Ophthalmol* 1991;112:623–631.
168. Uemura A: New inferior retinal detachment after scleral buckling procedure with intraocular gas injection. *Jpn J Ophthalmol* 1992;36:426–435.
169. Tornambe PE, Grizzard WS (eds): *Pneumatic Retinopexy: A Clinical Symposium.* Des Plaines, IL: Greenwood Publishing, 1989, p 173.
170. Lincoff H, Horowitz J, Kreissig I, et al: Morphological effect of gas compression on the cortical vitreous. *Arch Ophthalmol* 1986;104:1212–1215.
171. Panessa-Warren B, Maisel JM, Warren J: Alterations in rabbit vitreal fine structure following C_3F_8 injection. *Graefes Arch Clin Exp Ophthalmol* 1990;228: 541–551.
172. Constable IJ, Swann D: Vitreous substitutes, in Pruett RC, Regan CD (eds): *Retina Congress.* East Norwalk, CT: Appleton-Century-Crofts, 1971, pp 709–713.
173. Sebag J, Tang M: Pneumatic retinopexy using only air. *Retina* 1993;13:8–12.
174. McDonald HR, Abrams GW, Irvine AR, et al: The management of subretinal gas following attempted pneumatic retinal reattachment. *Ophthalmology* 1987;94: 319–326.
175. Wong D, Ansons AM, Chiynell AH, et al: Subretinal gas. *Eye* 1990;4:469–472.
176. Yeo JH, Vidaurri-Leal J, Glaser BM: Extension of retinal detachments as a complication of pneumatic retinopexy. *Arch Ophthalmol* 1986;104:1161–1163.
177. Hilton GF, Tornambe PE, Brinton DA, et al: The complications of pneumatic retinopexy. *Trans Am Ophthalmol Soc* 1990;88:191–210.
178. Speaker MG, Menikoff JA: Prophylaxis of endophthalmitis with topical povidone-iodine. *Ophthalmology* 1991;98:1769–1775.
179. Isenberg SJ, Apt L, Yoshimori R, et al: Chemical preparation of the eye in ophthalmic surgery: IV. Comparison of povidone-iodine on the conjunctiva with a prophylactic antibiotic. *Arch Ophthalmol* 1985;103:1340–1342.
180. Apt L, Isenberg S, Yoshimori R, et al: Chemical preparation of the eye in ophthalmic surgery: III. Effect of povidone-iodine on the conjunctiva. *Arch Ophthalmol* 1984;102:728–729.
181. Steinmetz RL, Kreiger AE, Sidikaro Y: Previtreous space gas sequestration during pneumatic retinopexy. *Am J Ophthalmol* 1989;107:191–192.
182. Meyers SM, FitzGibbon EJ: Simultaneous external subretinal fluid drainage and intravitreal gas injection. *Arch Ophthalmol* 1985;103:1881–1883.

183. Peyman GA, Paylor RR: Simultaneous perfusion of air and irrigating solution in the management of traumatic posterior segment injuries. *Retina* 1986;6:151–153.
184. Brucker AJ, Hoffman ME, Navyas HJ, et al: New instrumentation for fluid–air exchange. *Retina* 1985;3:135–136.
185. Freeman HM, Schepens CL, Couvillion GC: Current management of giant retinal breaks. *Trans Am Acad Ophthalmol Otolaryngol* 1970;74:59–74.
186. Cairns JD, Campbell WG: Vitrectomy techniques in the treatment of giant retinal tears: A flexible approach. *Aust N Z J Ophthalmol* 1988;16:209–214.
187. Holland PM, Smith TR: Broad scleral buckle in the management of retinal detachments with giant tears. *Am J Ophthalmol* 1977;83:518–525.
188. Wessing A, Spitznas M, Palomar A: Management of retinal detachments due to giant tears. *Albrecht von Graefes Arch Klin Ophthalmol* 1974;192:277–284.
189. Machemer R, Allen AW: Retinal tears 180° and greater: Management with vitrectomy and intravitreal gas. *Arch Ophthalmol* 1976;94:1340–1346.
190. Freeman HM, Couvillion GC, Schepens CL: Vitreous surgery: IV. Intraocular balloon: Clinical application. *Arch Ophthalmol* 1970;83:715–721.
191. Cibis PA: Vitreous transfer and silicone injections. *Trans Am Acad Ophthalmol Otolaryngol* 1964;68:983–997.
192. Fitzgerald CR: The use of Healon® in a case of rolled-over retina. *Retina* 1981;1:227–231.
193. Schepens CL, Marden D: Data on the natural history of retinal detachment: Further characterization of certain unilateral nontraumatic cases. *Am J Ophthalmol* 1966;61:213–226.
194. Schepens CL, Freeman HM: Current management of giant retinal breaks. *Trans Am Acad Ophthalmol Otolaryngol* 1967;71:474–487.
195. Amoils SP: *Cryosurgery in Ophthalmology.* Chicago: Year Book, 1975, pp 162–165.
196. Peyman GA, Rednam KRV, Seetner AA: Retinal microincarceration with penetrating diathermy in the management of giant retinal tears. *Arch Ophthalmol* 1984;102:562–565.
197. Howard RO, Gaasterland DE: Giant retinal dialysis and tear: Surgical repair. *Arch Ophthalmol* 1970;84:312–315.
198. Galezowski X: Du décollement de la rétine, et de son traitement. *Bull Mem Soc Fr Ophtalmol* 1889;7:200–202.
199. Heimann K: Zur Behandlung komplizierter Riesenrisse der Netzhaut. *Klin Monatsbl Augenheilkd* 1980;176:491–492.
200. Federman JL, Shakin JL, Lanning RC: The microsurgical management of giant retinal tears with trans-scleral retinal sutures. *Ophthalmology* 1982;89:832–839.
201. Scott JD: A new approach to the vitreous base. *Mod Probl Ophthalmol* 1974;12:407–410.
202. Usui M, Hamazaki S, Takano S, et al: A new surgical technique for the treatment of giant tear: Transvitreoretinal fixation. *Jpn J Ophthalmol* 1979;23:206–215.
203. Hirose T, Schepens CL, Lopansri C: Subtotal open-sky vitrectomy for severe retinal detachment occurring as a late complication of ocular trauma. *Ophthalmology* 1981;88:1–9.
204. Kreissig I, Lincoff H, Stanowsky A: The treatment of giant tear detachments using retrohyaloidal perfluorocarbon gases without drainage or vitrectomy. *Graefes Arch Clin Exp Ophthalmol* 1987;225:94–98.

205. Brown GC, Benson WE: Use of sodium hyaluronate for the repair of giant retinal tears. *Arch Ophthalmol* 1989;107:1246–1249.
206. Peyman GA, Smith RT: Use of fluorosilicone to unfold a giant retinal tear. *Int Ophthalmol* 1987;10:149–151.
207. Grizzard WS, Hammer ME: A simplified approach to treating retinal detachment from giant retinal tears. *Vitreoretinal Surg Technol* 1989;1(2):1,3,5.
208. Hoffman ME, Sorr EM: Management of giant retinal tears without scleral buckling. *Retina* 1986;6:197–204.
209. Gnad H, Paroussis P, Skorpik C: An intraocular balloon for silicone oil implantation. *Graefes Arch Clin Exp Ophthalmol* 1986;224:18–20.
210. Glaser BM: Treatment of giant retinal tears combined with proliferative vitreoretinopathy. *Ophthalmology* 1986;93:1193–1197.
211. Joondeph BC, Flynn HW Jr, Blankenship GW, et al: The surgical management of giant retinal tears with the cannulated extrusion needle. *Am J Ophthalmol* 1989;108:548–553.
212. Glaser BM. Treatment of giant tears combined with proliferative vitreoretinopathy, in Ryan SJ (ed): *Retina*, vol. 3, *Surgical Retina*. St. Louis: CV Mosby, 1989, pp 449–454.
213. Joondeph BC, Blankenship GW: Hemostatic effects of air versus fluid in diabetic vitrectomy. *Ophthalmology* 1989;96:1701–1706.
214. Williams DF, Peters MA, Abrams GW, et al: A two-stage technique for intraoperative fluid–gas exchange following pars plana vitrectomy. *Arch Ophthalmol* 1990;108:1484–1486.
215. Worsley DR, Grey RHB: Supplemental gas tamponade after conventional scleral buckling surgery: A simple alternative to surgical revision. *Br J Ophthalmol* 1991; 75:535–537.
216. Topping TM: Discussion: Hemostatic effects of air versus fluid in diabetic vitrectomy by BC Joondeph and GW Blankenship. *Ophthalmology* 1989;96:1706–1707.

Chapter 3
Perfluorocarbon Liquids

PERFLUOROCARBON LIQUIDS: BACKGROUND AND GENERAL CONSIDERATIONS

For more than three decades, lighter-than-water vitreous substitutes such as silicone[1-10] and gas[11-16] have played an important role in the management of complicated retinal detachments, both intraoperatively as a surgical tool and postoperatively by exerting a short- or long-term tamponading effects on the retina. As intraocular tamponading agents, they keep the retina in contact with the underlying retinal pigment epithelium (RPE) until the chorioretinal scars that form in areas of retinal tears are strong enough to prevent retinal detachment. Although these substances exert some degree of pressure on the upper part of the retina, the loss of support in the inferior part of the vitreous cavity causes accumulation of fluid with subsequent membrane formation in this area. Thus, inferior tractional retinal detachments are often seen with the use of low-specific-gravity silicone oil.[5,10,17,18]

Heavier-than-water vitreous substitutes include fluorosilicone oil and perfluorocarbon liquids (PFCLs). Intraocular toxicity and high viscosity limit the use of fluorosilicone as a vitreous substitute and internal tamponading agent.

Perfluorocarbons are hydrocarbons in which fluorine atoms have chemically replaced hydrogen atoms. At room temperature, those with more than six carbon atoms are liquid, whereas those with fewer than four carbon atoms are gases. Perfluorocarbon gases are widely used in vitreoretinal surgery.

Perfluorocarbon liquids are fully fluorinated, man-made compounds containing carbon–fluorine bonds. These organic liquids are composed of both high- and low-molecular-weight polymers. Because they possess an extensive capacity for transporting and releasing both O_2 and CO_2, PFCLs were initially developed by Clark and Gollan[19] as blood substitutes capable of providing gas transport functions in both animals and humans,[19-21] and they are currently used during coronary angioplasty to deliver oxygen to ischemic myocardial tissue.[22-24] Liquid perfluorocarbons have had a variety of uses in medicine as blood substitutes, in the preservation of organs for transplantation, and as diagnostic aids with imaging techniques.[19-24] PFCLs with a viscosity near that of water have been considered generally biologically inert.[19,25] No human enzyme system is capable of breaking down these compounds metabolically.

Toxicity in PFCLs is frequently caused by small amounts of unsaturated hydrogen-containing compounds. Among impurities found in PFCLs are small amounts of compounds with N–F bonds, which cause the greatest toxicity, and unsaturated hydrogen-containing compounds, which are also toxic.[26] Purification of PFCLs requires removal of these compounds.[26] H-Nucleic magnetic resonance (HNMR) and infrared (IR) spectroscopy and cell cultures can be used to determine the presence of these compounds in PFCLs.[27]

Low-viscosity perfluorocarbons are optically clear, with a specific gravity of 1.8 to 2.03. This characteristic allows the PFCLs to be used for hydrokinetic manipulation of the retina during vitrectomy. The specific gravity of PFCLs is almost double that of water, allowing the PFCLs to displace subretinal fluid and blood in the posterior pole anteriorly, negating the need for posterior drainage. PFCLs allow membrane dissection while stabilizing the posterior retina, thus diminishing the possibility of iatrogenic damage. No special contact lenses are required during surgery because the indices of refraction of these liquids are only slightly different from saline, and the low viscosity of the PFCL allows easy intraocular injection and removal.[28-38]

In 1966, Clark and Gollan[19] reported on the use of fluorocarbon liquids as oxygen transporters and blood substitutes. They demonstrated that mice immersed for 1 hour in a liquid perfluorocarbon equilibrated with oxygen at atmospheric pressure could survive by breathing this oxygenated liquid (Fig. 3–1).

Having suffered from a retinal detachment himself, Clark was aware of the potential importance of the various PFCLs for treatment of a detached retina, both as intraoperative tools and as postoperative vitreous replacement materials. He believed that "these compounds, having specific gravities greater than one, can be ideally employed in the treatment of retinal tears or detachments."[26] He found that when injected into the eye over the anterior surface of the retina, the "dense liquid, by means of gravity, will then compress the detached retina enabling retinal reattachment."[26] Because these liquids are heavier than water, the procedure could be performed with the patient lying on his back and the physician standing or sitting in a normal manner, thus avoiding the awkward positioning previously required for both patient and surgeon during surgery and for the patient during recovery. Furthermore, "the novel liquids may simply be removed after the retina is attached, if desired."[26]

Haidt et al,[39] in 1982, first experimentally evaluated the use of liquid perfluorocarbon as a vitreous substitute. In 1984, Zimmerman and Faris[40] reported the use of PFCLs (N-perfluorocarbon amines) as intraoperative tools for repositioning experimentally detached retinas.[40] Retinal detachments were produced by making inferior retinal breaks; the retina was then held in place by the perfluoroamines. In 1986, after joining Cornell University, Neal Zimmerman collaborated with Chang[41] in evaluating the intraoperative use of perfluorotributylamine. Miyamoto et al[28,42] evaluated the use of perfluoroether and other fluorinated compounds as experimental vitreous substitutes and concluded that these compounds were not suitable for long-term vitreous replacement. In 1989, Nabih et al[32] demonstrated that perfluoroperhydrophenanthrene was tolerated in the rabbit eye as a vitreous substitute.

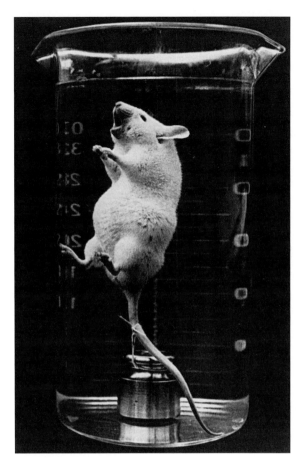

Figure 3–1. Submersed for 1 hour, mouse survives without air by breathing a liquid per-fluorocarbon equilibrated with oxygen.

Fluorinated hydrocarbons[28,29,30,36,42-46] have a specific gravity 1.7 to 2.03 times greater than water, which gives them a number of important characteristics. These liquids force subretinal fluid and blood anteriorly, eliminating the need to create a retinotomy for posterior drainage. The higher-than-water specific gravity allows the surgeon to use PFCLs for relatively atraumatic manipulation of the retina. PFCLs are used to unfold the retina in giant retinal tears. A small amount of PFCL injected intravitreally provides countertraction and retinal stabilization during membrane dissection in proliferative vitreoretinopathy (PVR). When adequate membrane dissection has been performed, PFCLs flatten the posterior retina or define further areas of traction that require elimination before the retina flattens. These substances eliminate the need for tacks or cyanoacrylates to fixate the retina after creation of the retinotomy.[33]

Internal tamponading agents should have high interfacial surface tension in water. High surface tension implies that the substance has strong cohesive characteristics, allowing internal closure of a retinal break while preventing the substance from flowing through a retinal tear into the subretinal space.[30,46,47]

Perfluorocarbons and silicone oil have nearly equivalent surface tensions (between 16 and 20 dynes/cm^2).[46] The internal tamponade exerted by fluorocarbon liquids is greater than that provided by an equivalent volume of fluorosilicone oil.[31] A transretinal force of 0.25 g is exerted by a 0.3-mL perfluorocarbon bubble, whereas a 1.0-mL bubble of silicone oil exerted an upward transretinal force of 0.06.[48] Sparrow et al[48] suggest that the transretinal force of a tamponading agent may be a more important factor than surface tension in determining the ability of an intraocular tamponading agent to resist tractional retinal detachment.

Perfluorocarbon liquids are also less viscous than silicone oil, and some are less viscous than water. Their viscosity ranges from 0.8 to 8.0 centistokes (cSt).[43] The low viscosity allows injection through 20- to 30-gauge needles. These liquids are easily removed from the eye using a 20-gauge flute needle.[29,33,36]

By keeping the tip of the needle inside the PFCL bubble during injection, the PFCL will remain as a single bubble inside the eye.[33] The index of refraction is also close to that of saline (1.28 to 1.33).[31] Thus, PFCLs can be identified during injection into a water-filled eye.[31]

Perfluorocarbon liquids are immiscible with blood. If bleeding occurs during surgery, the surgeon's view is not obscured as much in the presence of intravitreal fluorocarbon liquids as in a saline-filled eye.[36]

Sparrow and associates[48] evaluated the surface reactivity of alumina-treated PFCLs to assess the suitability of these compounds for use as vitreous substitutes. They were able to evaluate the inertness of these compounds by correlating the results with surface reactivity.

Table 3–1 describes most PFCLs used in ophthalmology and their characteristics.

TABLE 3–1. Perfluorocarbon Liquids

Perfluorocarbon	Chemical Formula	Specific Gravity	Viscosity (cSt, 25°C)	Refractive Index	Vapor Pressure (mm Hg at 37°C)	Surface Tension (dyne/cm)
Perfluorotributylamine	$C_{12}F_{27}N$	1.89	2.6	1.29	1.14	16
Perfluorooctane	C_8F_{18}	1.76	0.8	1.27	50	14
Perfluorooctylbromide	$C_8F_{17}Br$	1.93	2.3	1.30	1.1	18.2
Perfluorodecalin	$C_{10}F_{18}$	1.94	2.7	1.31	13.5	16
Perfluoroethylcyclohexane	C_2F_6	1.83	0.94	1.29	55	
Vitreon (Perfluoroperhydrophenanthrene)	$C_{14}F_{24}$	2.03	8.03	1.33	<1	18

INTRAOCULAR TOXICITY OF PFCLS

Using highly purified fluorocarbon liquids, Haidt and associates[39] replaced vitreous, aqueous, and other structures in cat, rabbit, and owl monkey eyes in 1982. After 3 months, some indications of ocular toxicity were found in eyes receiving a perfluorinated polymeric ether. Leakage from the site of injection was common, and all tested fluorocarbons produced "fish-egging." Several of the liquids, however, were well tolerated over several months, without corneal decompensation, changes in intraocular pressure (IOP), or cataracts. When *perfluoromethyldecalin* partially replaced the aqueous and vitreous in the eye of an owl monkey, no signs of toxicity were found.

Zimmerman and Faris[40] used a PFCL (*N-perfluorocarbon amine*) as an intraoperative tool for repositioning experimentally detached retinas without sign of toxicity.

Several experimental studies have demonstrated poor long-term tolerance of many PFCLs when left in the vitreous cavity.[28,31,41,42,49] Miyamoto et al evaluated two separate perfluoroether liquids, *Freon E15*[28] and *Fomblin-H Fluorinated Fluid*,[42] and found both substances to be unsuitable vitreous substitutes because of poor ocular tolerance. Bubbles and precipitates were found 1 month after injection in eyes receiving Freon E15, and by six months, preretinal membranes, retinal disorganization, and tractional retinal detachment were seen.[28] Preretinal membranes, retinal disorganization, and retinal detachment were also found by 6 months in eyes intravitreally injected with Fomblin.[42]

Chang and Zimmerman[41] evaluated the toxicity of intravitreal *perfluorotributylamine* ($C_{12}F_{27}N$). Studying 38 rabbit eyes over a period of up to 5 months, they concluded that the substance is a poor long-term vitreous substitute because of the dispersion, foam cell response, and photoreceptor toxicity if the retina was exposed to this substance for periods longer than 2 weeks. However, they stated that this PFCL provided a mechanical tamponade of the retina in eyes with experimental retinal detachment and that it did not escape through iatrogenic retinal breaks because of its interfacial tension. The retinal changes did not occur if the PFCL was removed after the second day. As suggested by Clark,[26] Chang and associates[45] advocated intraoperative use of PFCLs as a surgical tool.

Chang and associates[50] demonstrated histopathologically a lack of retinal toxicity when *perfluoro-n-octane* liquid was left in the vitreous cavity of pig eyes for 3 hours. These investigators preferred perfluoro-n-octane over other PFCLs because it has a lower boiling point and higher vapor pressure (approximately 50 mm Hg at 37°C[51]) than the other two perfluorocarbons. Small intravitreal residual volumes (0.1 mL) of perfluoro-n-octane were well tolerated for at least 6 months.[50]

Velikay et al,[49] in an experimental study in rabbits, compared highly purified perfluorodecalin and nonpurified perfluorodecalin for long-term vitreous replacement.

The experiment involved purified perfluorodecalin of 95% to 98% purity, which underwent an additional chemical procedure for further purification, and perfluorodecalin, which was not specially purified. All substances were sterilized by filtering twice through a 0.22-μm Millipore filter. In control eyes, the vitreous was replaced with lactated Ringer's solution. One week after surgery, there was no difference in inflammation between eyes with highly purified decalin and control eyes. Narrowing of the retinal vessels was noted in all eyes given decalin. Microaneurysms of retinal vessels occurred in one third of the eyes, regardless of the substance used. Intravitreal fibrin membranes developed in two thirds of the eyes with unpurified decalin. Foam cells and intraretinal macrophages were observed in all eyes receiving this PFCL.[49]

After 2 weeks, a necrosis of the retina at the interface of the PFCL and the aqueous was observed. After 4 weeks, interface necrosis was seen in all eyes with perfluorodecalin. In the third and fourth postoperative weeks, 8 of the 10 eyes with unpurified perfluorodecalin developed retinal detachments; all retinas stayed attached in the group with the highly purified PFCL. After 8 weeks, the severity of the lesions in the eyes with highly purified perfluorodecalin had increased, and the retina had developed localized areas in which photoreceptors were missing or localized areas of atrophy of all layers of the retina in the lower part of the eye. All layers of the retina in the upper part of the eye showed thinning and vacuolization of the ganglion cell layer and inner nuclear layer.[49]

Velikay and co-workers[49] concluded that physical and chemical properties of the PFCLs other than specific gravity alone are important in retinal tolerance of vitreous substitutes. Also, the degree of purification of the PFCL had an impact on the histopathologic changes caused by mechanical stress. The toxic effect of impurities was also indicated by the rate of retinal detachment in eyes treated with nonpurified decalin.[49]

Eckardt and associates[52] compared the intraocular toxicity of *perfluorooctane* and two *perfluoropolyethers* injected intraocularly in rabbit eyes after pars plana vitrectomy. Histologic examination of eyes 8 hours postinjection showed no short-term intraocular toxicity for any of these three PFCLs. Perfluorooctane- and perfluoropolyether-injected eyes postoperatively demonstrated major retinal morphologic changes at 6 days to 2 months. These abnormalities were primarily confined to the lower retina, which is an area where permanent contact with the perfluorocarbon is maintained.

Perfluorooctylbromide (PFOB) was developed initially as a radiological contrast medium and has been used as an imaging agent in magnetic resonance imaging (MRI), computed tomography (CT), ultrasound, and conventional radiography.[53-55] Initial ophthalmic evaluation of PFOB was reported by Flores-Aguilar et al,[56] who found it to be nontoxic to the retina when used as an intraoperative tool in rabbits.

Conway et al[57] studied the toxicity of *perfluorooctylbromide* as a short-term postoperative vitreous substitute in African green monkeys. After vitrectomy and vitreous replacement with 1.5 to 2.0 mL of PFOB, lenses remained clear in all eyes, although in the immediate postoperative period, one eye became inflamed and had a culture-negative vitritis. The other eyes showed a minimal anticipated postoperative vitreous inflammation. Emulsification of the PFOB began within 3 days of injection and progressed up to 3 weeks, precluding fundus examination and fluorescein angiography in 2 weeks. Eyes were enucleated and light microscopy performed at 2,

10, 33, and 45 days. Indirect examination was normal up to 10 days; thereafter, the fundus view was obscured by the emulsified PFOB.

After 45 days, the cornea had a mixed cellular inflammatory reaction on the corneal endothelium (Fig. 3–2A). On histologic examination of this eye, a few cells were noted in the anterior chamber angle. Globules of PFOB admixed with inflammatory cells were adherent to the posterior surface of the lens capsule; this explained the posterior lenticular opacity seen clinically (Fig. 3–2B). Globules of PFOB lined the surface of the ciliary body and the retina. There was evidence of preretinal cellular debris at 10, 33, and 45 days. Retinal perivasculitis was seen at 33 and 45 days

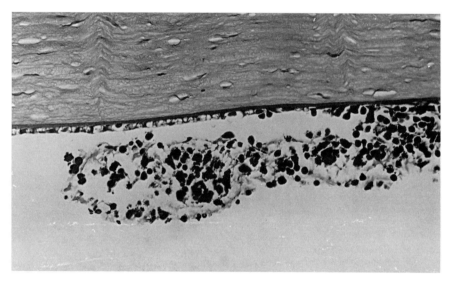

A

Figure 3–2. Use of perfluorooctylbromide (PFOB) as a vitreous substitute in African green monkeys. **A.** Cornea 45 days after instillation of PFOB into vitreous cavity. Note inflammatory cells and fibrin adherent to endothelium (× 450). **B.** Posterior surface of crystalline lens 45 days after instillation of PFOB into vitreous cavity. Inflammatory cells and globules of PFOB can be seen on posterior surface of lens capsule (× 650). **C.** Retina 45 days after injection of PFOB into vitreous cavity. There is marked perivasculitis (large arrow) surrounding this retinal vessel and vacuolization of surrounding retinal structures. Globules of PFOB and inflammatory cellular debris are seen in preretinal vitreous (small arrow). (From Conway MD, Peyman GA, Karaçorlu M, et al: Perfluorooctylbromide (PFOB) as a vitreous substitute in non-human primates. *Int Ophthalmol* 1993;17:259–264. Reprinted by permission of Kluwer Academic Publishers.)

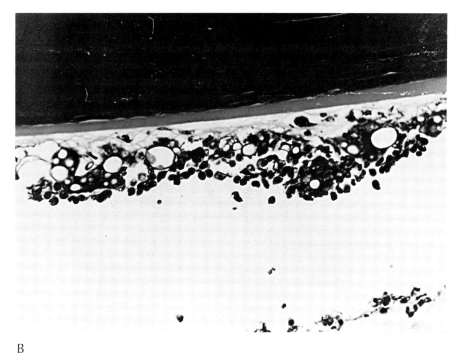

B

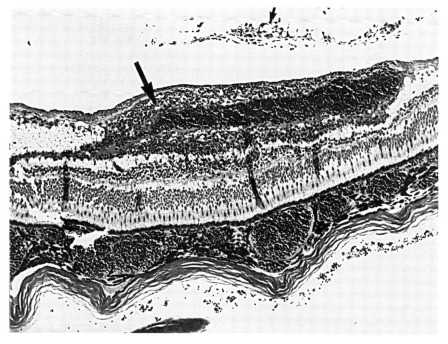

C

Figure 3–2 (Continued).

(Fig. 3–2C). PFOB seemed most suitable for intraoperative rather than postoperative use.

Perfluoroethylcyclohexane is a high-vapor-pressure PFCL (approximately 55 mm Hg at 37°C). Sparrow et al[51] evaluated retinal tolerance to intravitreal perfluoroethylcyclohexane. They injected the substance into eight rabbit eyes and allowed it to remain there for 48 hours. Electroretinography (ERG) and histologic studies performed up to 2 months after removal showed amplitudes and morphologic features comparable with those found in control eyes.

An additional 39 rabbit eyes underwent long-term intravitreal placement of perfluoroethylcyclohexane for periods ranging from 1 to 8 weeks. The researchers found that when perfluoroethylcyclohexane was allowed to remain intravitreally for more than 1 week, the liquid dispersed, and macrophages accumulated in front of the retina. Outer segments of photoreceptors were distorted and the outer plexiform layer narrowed.

Four eyes, which were not vitrectomized, received injections comparable to the quantity of perfluoroethylcyclohexane that might remain residually after PFCL removal. No histologic changes were found when such amounts were left in the eye up to 6 months.

In contrast to the results of studies on other PFCLs, experimental[35] and clinical studies[33,38,58,59] suggest that *perfluoroperhydrophenanthrene* (Vitreon, Vitrophage, Inc., Lyons, IL) may be used as a short-term postoperative intraocular tamponade to hold the retina in place until chorioretinal adhesions formed by laser photocoagulation or cryopexy are adequately developed to prevent redetachment. Although corneal damage was demonstrated after injection of perfluoroperhydrophenanthrene into the anterior chamber of experimental eyes,[58] such damage was not attributed by the investigators to the toxic effects of perfluoroperhydrophenanthrene, but rather to mechanical damage resulting from contact of the perfluoroperhydrophenanthrene with corneal endothelial cells.

Experimental studies demonstrated this PFCL (Fig. 3–3) to have no toxic effect on tissue culture–grown cells and to be tolerated in vitrectomized rabbit eyes when left in place for 6 weeks.[32] No acute toxic or inflammatory reactions were noted intraoperatively or in the immediate postoperative period. In rabbit eyes, fragmentation of the perfluoroperhydrophenanthrene into small globules in the vitreous cavity was noted at 6 weeks, which is later in onset than previously studied liquid perfluorocarbons.[41] Postoperative ERG recordings disclosed no pathologic changes in eyes tested. Light and electron microscopy of eyes of rabbits killed at the end of follow-up showed retention of normal retinal architecture with no evidence of retinal toxicity. Corneal toxicity as evidenced by corneal edema was noted, however, after injection of perfluoroperhydrophenanthrene into the anterior chamber of rabbit eyes.

In another study,[35] African green monkeys underwent vitrectomy and vitreous replacement with perfluoroperhydrophenanthrene or perfluoroperhydrophenanthrene plus silicone oil. Perfluoroperhydrophenanthrene alone and in combination with silicone remained optically clear and allowed fundus examination up to 162 days (Fig. 3–4A–J). No toxic effects to the retina were detectable. Medical-grade silicone with a viscosity of 10 cSt was used. Emulsification of perfluoroperhy-

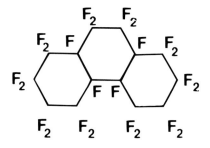

$$C_{14}F_{24}$$

Figure 3–3. Chemical structures of perfluoroperhydrophenanthrene.

drophenanthrene started at approximately 72 days, with a few small granules appearing on the retinal surface. Emulsification progressed to involve the posterior vitreous cavity over the next 72 days, followed by an apparent decrease. The fundus, including retinal detail and vessels, was clearly visible despite the emulsification. Vitreon and silicone failed to migrate into the anterior chamber in any eye and, with the exception of one eye with a traumatic cataract, all lenses remained clear. Electron microscopy performed at 45, 98, and 162 days demonstrated normal retinal architecture. At 162 days postinjection, one eye with perfluoroperhydrophenanthrene, one eye with perfluoroperhydrophenanthrene plus silicone, and a control eye demonstrated normal ERGs and normal intravenous fluorescein angiograms (Fig. 3–4E–F).

Perfluoroperhydrophenanthrene contains inherent physical properties necessary for a desirable denser-than-water temporary vitreous substitute. It has a specific gravity of 2.03, a viscosity of 8.03 cSt, and a boiling point of 215°C. It is immiscible with water, optically clear, radiopaque (Fig. 3–5), easily injected and removed through a small (20- to 25-gauge) needle. Its low vapor pressure (>1 mm Hg at 37°C) permits air travel without the danger of gas formation in the eye.

Preliminary clinical studies by Peyman et al[36] and Blinder et al[33] demonstrated that perfluoroperhydrophenanthrene could be left in the eye for up to 28 days as a temporary tamponading agent without any evidence of intraocular toxicity. Perfluoroperhydrophenanthrene did not emulsify in any of these eyes; after removal it was replaced by gas, air, or silicone.

The fluorinated hydrocarbons used by Zimmerman and Faris[40] and by Chang et al[45,50] require immediate removal at the end of surgery to prevent retinal toxicity. However, perfluoroperhydrophenanthrene can be used intraoperatively and kept inside the eye in the postoperative period, eliminating the need for prone positioning of these patients (a major disadvantage of the previous methodology using gas or silicone oil).

Small perfluoroperhydrophenanthrene drops, which were seen in five patients in the postoperative period after intraoperative removal of perfluoroperhydrophenanthrene, did not cause any toxic effects in these patients. Retinal or

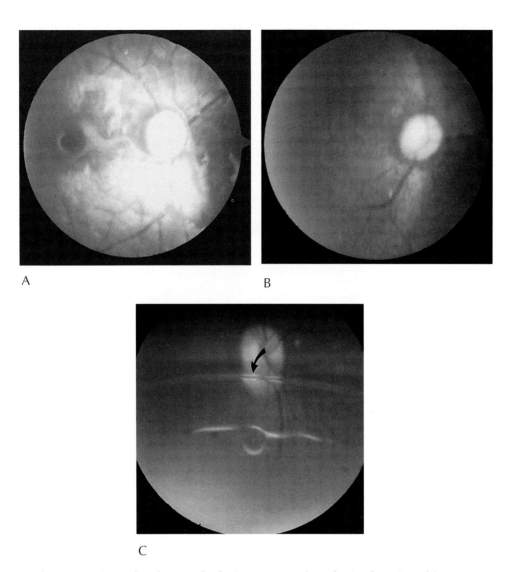

Figure 3–4. A. Fundus photograph of primate eye 75 days after implantation of the per-fluoroperhydrophenanthrene. The bright areas seen in the photo are light reflexes from the oily surface of the retina. **B.** Fundus photograph of primate eye 162 days after per-fluoroperhydrophenanthrene implantation. Note decreased fundus visibility. **C.** Fundus photograph of primate eye taken with animal in erect position. Note the meniscus (arrow) between the perfluoroperhydrophenanthrene and silicone in the midvitreous cavity. *(Figure continues)*

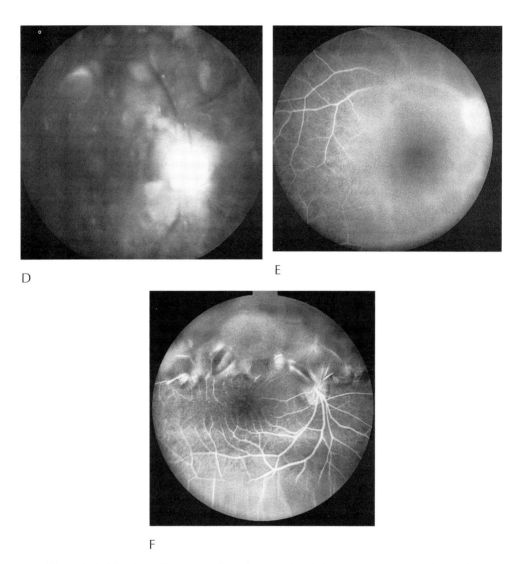

D

E

F

Figure 3–4 (Continued). D. Fundus photograph of the primate eye 98 days after implantation of perfluoroperhydrophenanthrene plus silicone. Photograph was taken with the animal in supine position. Note numerous silicone bubbles (arrows) obstructing the fundus view. **E.** Fluorescein angiogram of the primate eye shown in **B.** Note obstructed view of the retinal vessels at the area of perfluoroperhydrophenanthrene emulsification. There is no dye leakage from the visible retinal vessels. **F.** Fluorescein angiogram demonstrating obstructed view at the area of silicone emulsification. The fundus view through the perfluoroperhydrophenanthrene is unobstructed. Note that there is no leakage from the retinal vessels. *(Figure continues)*

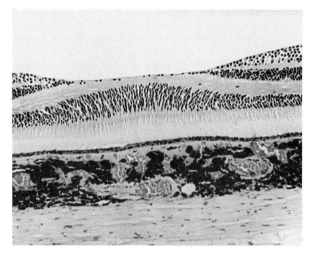

G

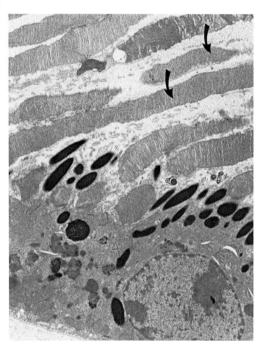

H

Figure 3–4 (Continued). G. Light micrograph of the monkey retina (foveal area, arrow) after 98 days of perfluoroperhydrophenanthrene plus silicone implantation. Note absence of preretinal membrane formation and cell infiltration in the vitreous. The retinal structures, including photoreceptor outer segments (curved arrows) appear normal. (HE, ×350.) **H.** Electron micrograph of the retinal outer structure 162 days after perfluoroperhydrophenanthrene implantation. Note normal structure of retinal pigment epithelium (RPE) and photoreceptor outer segments (arrows). (Uranyl acetate, × 5000.) *(Figure continues)*

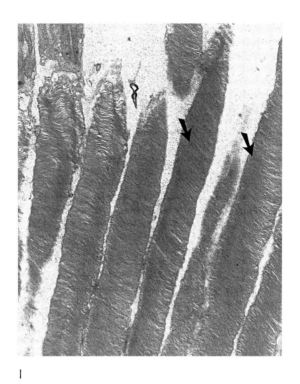

I

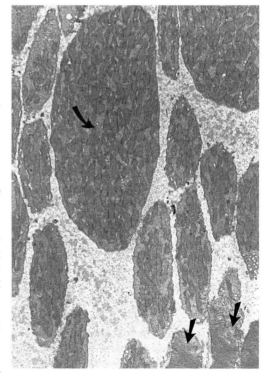

Figure 3–4 (Continued). I. Electron micrograph of the retinal outer structures 162 days after implantation with perfluoroperhydrophenanthrene. Note normal photoreceptor outer segments (arrows). (Uranyl acetate, × 10,000.) **J.** Electron micrograph of retinal outer structures 162 days after implantation with perfluoroperhydrophenanthrene. Note photoreceptor inner segment (curved arrows) packed with mitochondriae. Straight arrows point to normal outer segment. (Uranyl acetate, × 5000.) (From Peyman GA, Conway MD, Soike KF, et al: Long-term vitreous replacement in primates with intravitreal Vitreon or Vitreon plus silicone. *Ophthalmic Surg* 1991;22:657–664.)

J

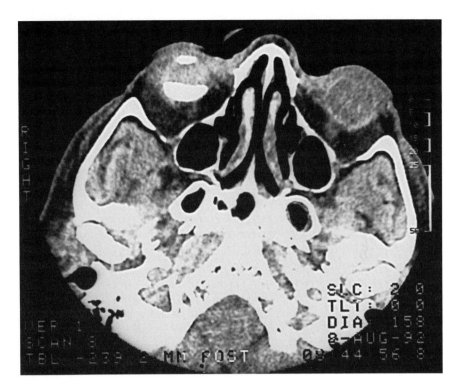

Figure 3–5. Perfluoroperhydrophenanthrene is radiopaque. (From Millsap CM, Peyman GA, Mehta NJ: Perfluoroperhydrophenanthrene (Vitreon) is radiopaque. *Ophthalmic Surg* 1993;24:500).

choroidal changes were not observed as a result of contact with the perfluoroperhydrophenanthrene droplets. The viscosity of perfluoroperhydrophenanthrene (8.03 cSt) and surface tension (18 dyne/cm^2) limit its passage through small posterior retinal holes.

No emulsification was observed of perfluoroperhydrophenanthrene left in the eye for as long as 28 days. Emulsification, however, was observed when perfluoroperhydrophenanthrene was implanted in the rabbit eye for a period of 6 weeks. The emulsification of the PFCL occurs as a result of changes in interfacial tension between the PFCL and the vitreous fluid, as has been seen in other artificial vitreous substitutes, such as low-viscosity silicone, fluorosilicone,[60] or other PFCLs.[50] The purity of the perfluoroperhydrophenanthrene used in this study might have played a role in the prevention of early emulsification.

Tanji and associates[59] reported on 41 consecutive eyes with complex vitreoretinal disease in which perfluoroperhydrophenanthrene was used as a postoperative tool and vitreous substitute. Postoperative use of perfluoroperhydrophenanthrene ranged from 3 days to 9 weeks, with a mean of 3.3 weeks. All retinas were attached intraoperatively, with a macular reattachment rate of 73% and an anatomic success rate of 100% after additional surgery. Cataract formation attributed to mechanical interference with normal metabolic exchange through the posterior capsule occurred in 50% of phakic eyes. Transient increased IOP was present in four eyes (10%) and persisted after perfluoroperhydrophenanthrene removal in only one eye. This single eye with persistent glaucoma had an inflammatory glaucoma before surgery. Additional postoperative complications included macular pucker, recurrent PVR, and anterior fibrinous reaction, which occurred at rates equal to or lower than those reported for vitreoretinal surgery without perfluoroperhydrophenanthrene.[61-63] No corneal complications occurred. In 80% of eyes, visual acuity either improved or remained stable. No toxic effects attributable to perfluoroperhydrophenanthrene were observed.

A multicenter clinical study by Greve et al[64] evaluated the efficacy of perfluoroperhydrophenanthrene in the management of complex retinal detachments and posteriorly dislocated lenses. Seven hundred patients underwent procedures using this substance as an intraoperative or short-term vitreous substitute.

The most common indications for the use of perfluoroperhydrophenanthrene included retinal detachment associated with proliferative PVR (282 patients, 40%); giant retinal tear with retinal detachment (94 patients, 13.4%); retinal detachment associated with a history of trauma (93 patients, 13.3%); and removal of a dislocated crystalline nucleus or intraocular lens (IOL) (41 patients, 6%). The most common postoperative complications were recurrent retinal detachment with or without PVR (79 patients, 11%); epiretinal membrane formation including macular pucker, 41 eyes (5.9%); fibrinous reaction in the vitreous cavity, 28 eyes (4%); residual perfluoroperhydrophenanthrene 27 eyes (3.8%); and vitreous hemorrhage, 18 eyes (2.6%). This study shows perfluoroperhydrophenanthrene to be an effective intraoperative tool that lacks toxicity when used as a short-term vitreous tamponade or to treat complex retinal detachment, PVR, expulsive hemorrhage, subluxated nucleus, and dislocated lens. It is also safe for several less common conditions, such as optic nerve coloboma associated with serous retinal detachment, retinal incarceration, and complicated cases of traumatic retinal detachment.

COMBINATIONS OF PERFLUOROCARBON LIQUID AND SILICONE OIL

Based on experimental studies using silicone oil in combination with the PFCL perfluoroperhydrophenanthrene, Peyman, Blinder, and associates[35,37] concluded that a combination of silicone oil (3 mL) and PFCL (0.5 mL) would take advantage of the greater ability of PFCLs to resist tractional retinal detachment and ensure that the interface between the two liquids could not involve the visual axis. Because of its lesser viscosity, silicone has less of a tendency to enter the anterior chamber of aphakic eyes than PFCLs and may restrict the movement of the PFCL into the anterior chamber.

Sparrow and associates[48] speculated that vitreous replacement with a mixture of silicone oil and PFCL in a 2:1 ratio might provide better resistance to the tractional forces complicating complex retinal detachments than either vitreous substitute might alone.

Experiments by Peyman and associates[35] and Blinder et al[33,37] also suggested that silicone oil tends to delay the emulsification of PFCLs when both substances are used together as vitreous replacements.

Clinical studies have demonstrated good tolerance of the combination of silicone and perfluoroperhydrophenanthrene used in the human eye.[33,64]

A potential problem with perfluorocarbons that are used in aphakic eyes as postoperative intraocular tamponading agents involves the entrance of the liquid into the anterior chamber. Moreira et al[65] injected 0.05 mL perfluoropolyether or perfluorooctane into the anterior chamber of rabbit eyes. External photography and biomicroscopy demonstrated corneal clouding and vascularized pannus formation along with conjunctival inflammation, anterior chamber flare, and the formation of small bubbles on the cornea called "fish-egging." The histopathology of trephined corneas after the animals were killed at 14 days showed vacuoles of PFCL present in the corneal endothelium but not in the stroma, retrocorneal inflammatory membranes, and an inflammatory ridge associated with damaged endothelial cells limited to the area of the cornea that was in contact with the PFCL.

Based on this corneal toxicity resulting from the presence of either of two PFCLs in the anterior chamber for 2 weeks, Moreira et al[65] caution against the short- or long-term use of perfluorocarbons as vitreous substitutes in aphakic eyes.

Subretinal PFCL has been reported as a complication of vitrectomy in eyes with complicated retinal detachment.

De Queiroz et al[66] determined the effect of subretinal PFCLs after vitrectomy and retinotomy in 26 rabbit eyes injected subretinally with 0.03 mL of either perfluorooctane or perfluorotributylamine. Before being killed, the animals were monitored by indirect ophthalmoscopy and fundus photography for intervals up to 21 days. Light-adapted ERGs were performed for up to 21 days. The retina remained flat, with a normal appearance, with the exception of a torn retinotomy site in three animals. ERG results were normal as compared with controls. Histology demonstrated degeneration or the absence of the photoreceptor outer segments only in areas where the retina was in contact with the PFCLs. No signs of retinal atrophy and mild inner nuclear edema were found. The investigators attributed the retinal changes to the mechanical rather than the toxic effects of the PFCLs. Because the same complications may occur in humans, De Queiroz et al[66] suggest removal of subretinal perfluorocarbon intraoperatively during the same vitrectomy session.

COMBINATION OF PFCL AND INTRAOCULAR GAS

The use of an intraocular gas with PFCLs has been suggested to provide both a superior and inferior tamponading effect that offers potential therapeutic advantages over the use of either vitreous substitute alone.

A rabbit model was used to evaluate the effect of intravitreal perfluoroperhydrophenanthrene on the decay rate of intraocular perfluoropropane (C_3F_8).[67] After gas displacement vitrectomy, one group of rabbit eyes was injected with 1.5 mL per-fluoroperhydrophenanthrene to give a 40% to 50% fill, and the control group received normal saline. Twenty-four hours later, 0.4 mL C_3F_8 was injected into all eyes. The average intraocular gas bubble expansion in the perfluoroperhy-drophenanthrene-filled eyes was 23%, compared with 80% in control eyes. The mean duration for total disappearance of the gas bubble was considerably shortened in the perfluoroperhydrophenanthrene-filled eye compared with the control (11 ± 3 versus 32 ± 5 days). IOP on day 1 postoperatively was higher in the control eyes than the perfluoroperhydrophenanthrene-filled eyes but was similar for the duration of the experiment.

The investigators concluded that eyes with intravitreal perfluoroperhy-drophenanthrene demonstrated accelerated decay of intraocular C_3F_8 compared with controls. The investigators suggest that intravitreal perfluoroperhydrophenanthrene alters the normal gas bubble expansion and resorption by interacting with C_3F_8 by either absorption or other physicochemical mechanisms. This elevated interaction may severely limit the clinical usefulness of C_3F_8 in eyes containing perfluoroper-hydrophenanthrene.[67]

COMPRESSION EFFECTS OF PERFLUOROCARBONS ON THE RETINA

Stolba and associates[68] evaluated the retinal toxicity of perfluoroperhydrophenan-threne in vitrectomized rabbit eyes. The animals were killed, and eyes were enucle-ated 1, 2, 4, or 8 weeks after vitrectomy and perfluoroperhydrophenanthrene injec-tion. Eyes examined 2 weeks after surgery had incipient signs of retinal damage. Those examined after 4 weeks demonstrated single bumplike protrusions in the pho-toreceptor layer and thinning in the outer plexiform layer in the inferior retina. After 8 weeks, the changes were more intense, and nuclear dropdown and irregularities of the retinal layers were observed. ERG findings, however, showed no change, other than transient c-wave reduction, which was attributed to trauma of surgery. Stolba and associates concluded that histologic retinal damage was less severe than in their studies of other PFCLs and that the changes were limited to the inferior half of the retina. In our opinion, because the rabbit retina lacks vascularization, it is more like-ly to be compressed by PFCLs than the primate and human retina. However, for tam-ponading of the inferior retina in patients, one needs only 0.5 to 0.7 mL of Vitreon, an amount that is less likely to generate the same compression effect as that used by Stolba et al (1.2 mL).[68]

INTRAVITREAL INJECTION AND REMOVAL OF PERFLUOROCARBON LIQUIDS

Perfluorocarbon liquids possess a number of important characteristics that make them particularly well suited to certain types of surgical procedures. They may be used as a temporary vitreous substitute in the management of complicated retinal detachments.[36] Because of the high specific gravity of PFCL, subretinal fluid and blood are forced anteriorly, eliminating the need to create a retinotomy for posterior drainage in eyes without preexisting posterior retinal tears. Perfluorocarbons may be used in the unfolding of giant retinal tears, with a flattening force 3 times greater than an equal volume of fluorosilicone, and they make excellent retinal tamponading agents.

Perfluorocarbon liquids are injected through a 20-gauge needle over the optic disc (Fig. 3–6A). The heavier-than-water liquid forces subretinal fluid anteriorly, where it escapes through a retinal hole. PFCL is removed using a flute needle or active aspiration through a 20-gauge blunt cannula, the tip of which is brought over the surface of the retina (Fig. 3–6B–E). Intermittent air and fluid exchange ensures removal of all the PFCL. In some cases, PFCL may be replaced with silicone (1,000 or 12,500 cSt) to maintain a long-term tamponading effect.

During the initial stages of a clinical study initiated by Peyman et al,[36] a unique problem was confronted. Fourteen patients had presented with rhegmatogenous retinal detachments with peripheral breaks. In these patients, perfluoroperhydrophenanthrene was used to "steam roll" the subretinal fluid from the posterior pole out through the anterior retinal tear (Fig. 3–7A–C). This effect was achieved simply by injecting the PFCL over the optic disc and observing the flattening effect as the PFCL level rose. However, on removal of the perfluoroperhydrophenanthrene, redetachment occurred in some cases as the liquid fluorocarbon level decreased. In these cases, subretinal fluid was pushed past the retinal tear by PFCL pressure in the periphery (Fig. 3–7B) and did not escape through the defect. On removal of the PFCL, the subretinal fluid simply shifted back to its posterior gravity-dependent position. To avoid this complication in subsequent cases, we performed a limited air–fluid exchange (Fig. 3–7C) before filling the vitreous cavity with PFCL, causing the air bubble to tamponade the retina anterior to the tear. PFCL injection over the optic disc was continued, slowly displacing the subretinal fluid out through the peripheral break, but not allowing it to go anterior to this point. Once the retina was flat, endolaser or cryotherapy was applied when necessary.

Perfluoroperhydrophenanthrene has been replaced with silicone for both optical and mechanical tamponading reasons. In these circumstances, a portion of the perfluoroperhydrophenanthrene in the vitreous cavity is replaced with silicone, which is injected through one of the sclerotomies while the perfluoroperhydrophenanthrene is removed through a posteriorly placed flute needle.

Instillation of silicone oil or PFCLs also has been used as an adjunct to vitreoretinal surgery for complex retinal detachments and giant retinal tears.[33,69,70] Peyman and Mehta[71] have designed a new instrument for simultaneous intravitreal infusion of silicone oil and removal of PFCL. The instrument (Fig. 3–8 A, B) consists of a tapering 18-gauge outer infusion tube, with a coaxial 20-gauge inner aspiration tube set in a standard vitrectomy handpiece. The outer tube has two 0.75-mm ports located on opposite sides and a single 0.5-mm port at the distal end of the intraocular portion. The infusion conduit is connected by polyethylene tubing to a 5-cc or 10-cc syringe, which can be filled with 100 to 300 cSt silicone oil. The aspiration conduit is connected to a linear aspiration unit.

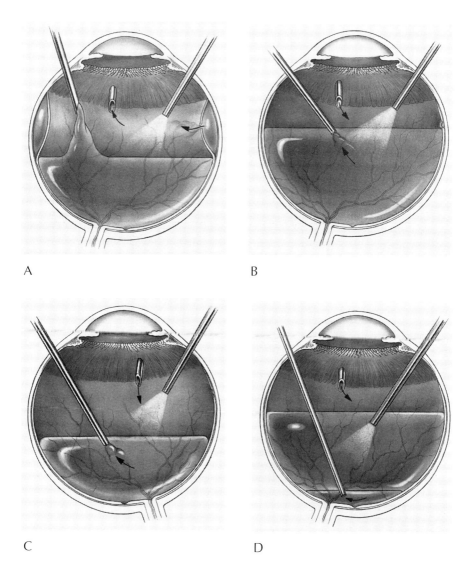

A   B

C   D

Figure 3–6. Schematic representation of the injection and removal of perfluoroperhy-drophenanthrene. **A.** Perfluoroperhydrophenanthrene is injected through a 20-gauge needle over the optic disc, forcing the subretinal fluid anteriorly, where it escapes through an anteriorly located retinal hole. **B.** Perfluoroperhydrophenanthrene is removed using a flute needle or active aspiration through a 20-gauge blunt cannula. **C.** Tip of cannula is brought over the surface of the retina. **D, E.** Intermittent air and fluid exchange ensures removal of all the perfluoroperhydrophenanthrene.

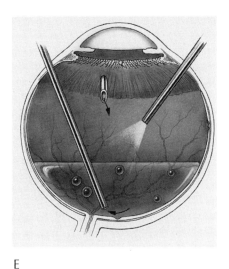

E

Figure 3–6 (Continued).

After completion of vitrectomy and membranectomy and reattachment of the retina with PFCL, one of the standard sclerotomies is enlarged to 3 mm to accommodate the 18-gauge handpiece. Silicone oil is then manually injected by an assistant while the surgeon aspirates the PFCL with the tip of the instrument held in the perfluorocarbon bubble until complete removal is obtained. The differences in refractive indices of silicone oil (1.40) and PFCLs allow for adequate visualization of the silicone–perfluorocarbon interface regardless of the type of PFCL used.[70] Complete removal can be ensured when silicone oil is aspirated at the end of the

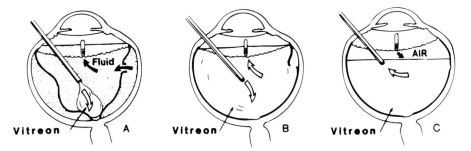

Figure 3–7. A–C. Use of perfluoroperhydrophenanthrene in patients with rhegmatogenous retinal detachments to "steam roll" the subretinal fluid from the posterior pole out through the anterior retinal tear. (From Blinder KJ, Peyman GA, Paris CL, et al: Vitreon, a new perfluorocarbon. *Br J Ophthalmol* 1991;75:240–244. By permission of Oxford University Press.)

exchange. This instrument can also be used to inject PFCL through the tip and remove infusion fluid through the side holes.

Visibility of PFCLs in a saline solution depends on several factors. One of these is the difference between the index of refraction of water (1.33) and that of PFCL. Except for perfluoroperhydrophenanthrene, which has an index of refraction of 1.33, PFCLs have a lower index of refraction than water. Therefore, the upper border of the perfluoroperhydrophenanthrene is more difficult to see in a physiologic saline solution than the borders of other PFCLs. However, in the vitreous cavity, small amounts of lipid, blood, or other particles in the liquid vitreous collect on the surface of the perfluoroperhydrophenanthrene, making its surface visible. In addition, the borders of a perfluoroperhydrophenanthrene-tamponaded retina remain attached compared with the detached peripheral retina, helping in localization of perfluoroperhydrophenanthrene. Hydrophobicity and surface tension cause small amounts of perfluoroperhydrophenanthrene to build a convex surface in the vitreous, making it slightly more visible than clear vitreous fluid. These phenomena aid the surgeon in seeing the borders of the perfluoroperhydrophenanthrene-filled cavity after only a few cases. As with air–fluid exchange, removal of perfluoroperhydrophenanthrene does not present a problem when air is used to replace Vitreon. However, an additional washout with saline ensures complete removal of PFCL.

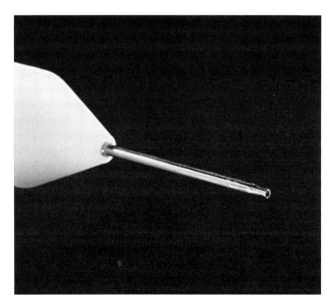

Figure 3–8. A. Intravitreal infusion-aspiration instrument. **B.** Schematic diagram of intraocular portion. Small arrows indicate path of silicone oil through infusion port. Large arrow points to perfluorocarbon-liquid aspiration tip. (From Peyman GA, Mehta NJ: Intravitreal infusion-aspiration instrument for silicone oil-perfluorocarbon liquid exchange. *Retina* 1993;13:177–178).

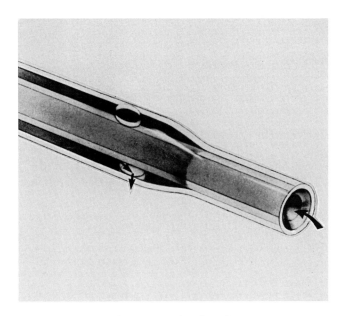

Figure 3–8 (Continued).

SPECIFIC TECHNIQUES USING PFCL

PFCLs in Giant Retinal Tear

Despite the advances in vitreoretinal surgery, repair of giant tears with PVR and a severely folded retina remains difficult. Even with the use of adjunct techniques involving silicone or air, manual attempts to unfold these retinal flaps are often unsuccessful.[72]

Perfluorocarbon liquid facilitates repair of a giant tear with the patient in a supine position. The PFCL fills the eye in a posterior-to-anterior direction when injected over the optic nerve. Intravitreal and subretinal fluids are forced anteriorly while the retina is hydrokinetically tamponaded against the RPE, preventing slippage. The need for drainage of subretinal fluid through a posterior retinotomy is obviated, thus eliminating potential complications from the retinotomy site, such as bleeding or membrane formation.[73]

Perfluorocarbon liquids can unfold even an extremely inverted retinal flap and hold it in place.

Endophotocoagulation is achieved more easily with the PFCLs, because subretinal fluid is removed completely,[33] minimizing dispersion of RPE cells.

Eyes with PVR and giant retinal tears also frequently present problems in management. After vitrectomy and membranectomy in these eyes, the intraoperative use of a small amount of PFCL allows the surgeon to determine whether all vitreous traction has been eliminated and the retina will completely flatten. Failure of the retina to flatten after intravitreal injection of PFCL suggests residual retinal traction.

The intraoperative use of a PFCL also provides countertraction and stabilization of the retina, facilitating membrane dissection.

Bottoni et al[74] used perfluorodecalin and postoperative supine positioning to manage 11 eyes with giant retinal tears and grade B PVR. After lensectomy and vitrectomy, perfluorodecalin was injected into the vitreous cavity. Patients were kept supine for 5 days, until a decalin–fluid exchange was performed in the operating room under general anesthesia. After a follow-up period of 18 months (range, 12 to 21 months), 9 (82%) of the 11 retinas were attached. Redetachment occurred in two eyes 15 days after surgery; a total of three reoperations were necessary to reattach the retinas. Functional improvement in visual acuity was achieved in the nine successfully reattached eyes; final visual acuity was 20/60 or better in eight eyes (89%) and 20/30 or better in seven (78%). No damage to the corneal endothelium was noted, because of supine positioning. However, perfluorodecalin has not been proven nontoxic to the retina.[49]

In the presence of unrelieved persistent traction caused by PVR, peripheral relaxing retinotomies[75-77] of varying degrees can be performed, followed by PFCL injection, to unroll, flatten, and stabilize the remaining posterior retina. The use of PFCL eliminates the need for retinal tacks[78-82] or cyanoacrylates[83] to fixate the retina during repair of giant tears intraoperatively or in the early postoperative period. In addition, the low viscosity of the PFCL permits its removal by passive egress through a flute needle during air–liquid exchange.

After vitrectomy and adequate removal of retinal traction, perfluoroperhydrophenanthrene is injected with a blunt 20-gauge to 27-gauge needle over the optic disk (Fig. 3–9A). The subretinal fluid is pushed in a posterior-to-anterior direction and out the giant retinal tear (Fig. 3–9B). When slippage of the retina occurs, the mechanical action of the PFCL elevates the retina into proper apposition with the RPE and unfolds the retinal flap of the giant tear. When the retina is completely flat, endolaser photocoagulation (Fig. 3–9C), cryopexy, or a combination of these procedures is performed. At this point, a decision is made either to replace the PFCL intraoperatively with sulfur hexafluoride (SF_6) (15% to 20%), C_3F_8 (10% to 15%), or silicone oil for a longer tamponading effect.

To remove PFCL from the eye, an air–PFCL exchange (Fig. 3–9D) is followed by three or four partial fluid–PFCL exchanges (Fig. 3–9E, F) to remove any residual PFCL. A silicone–air exchange is then performed, or the air–filled eyes are flushed with 25 cc 20% SF_6 or C_3F_8. An encircling scleral buckle can be placed.

Millsap et al[84] reported 50 patients with giant retinal tears managed with intraocular perfluoroperhydrophenanthrene. All patients were followed for at least 6 months, with a mean follow-up of 8.6 months. The area of the giant tear was less than 180° in 76% of patients, greater than 180° in 22%, and greater than 270° in 2%. PVR was present in 40%. In 84% of eyes, perfluoroperhydrophenanthrene was used only intraoperatively; in 16% it was left inside the eye for up to 4 weeks. Intraoperative retinal reattachment was achieved in 98% of eyes. Postoperative visu-

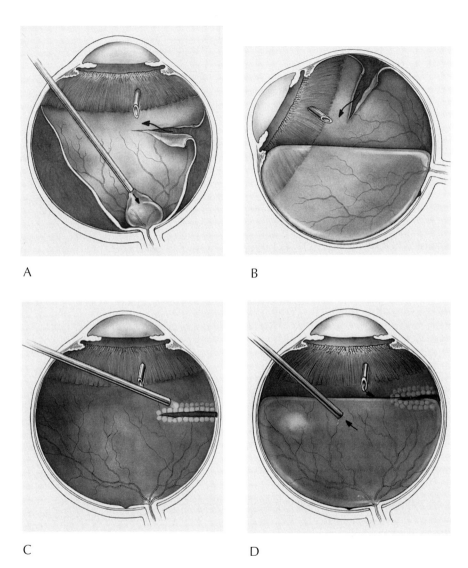

A

B

C

D

Figure 3–9. Management of giant retinal tears with intraocular perfluoroperhy-drophenanthrene. **A.** After vitrectomy, perfluoroperhydrophenanthrene is injected to flatten the detached retina. **B.** Posterior retina is attached as the perfluoroperhydro-phenanthrene fills the vitreous cavity. **C.** After complete attachment of the retina is achieved, endolaser photocoagulation is applied to the edge of the retinal tear. **D.** An air–perfluoroperhydrophenanthrene exchange is performed to remove most of the per-fluoroperhydrophenanthrene. **E.** A fluid–perfluoroperhydrophenanthrene exchange is performed to remove the remaining perfluoroperhydrophenanthrene. *(Figure continues)*

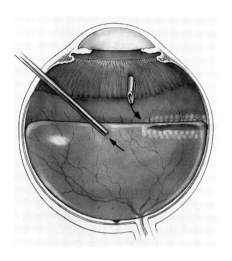

Figure 3–9 (Continued).   E

al acuity was better than 20/400 in 52%. Postoperative complications included cataract in 23%, choroidal effusion in 2%, hypotony in 4%, and recurrent retinal detachment with PVR in 26%. After an additional surgery, retinal attachment was achieved in 88% of all cases.

Our anatomic results compare well with results in three other series[52,85,86] where PFCLs were used to repair giant retinal tears. In previous series, the PFCL was removed intraoperatively in all eyes rather than being used as a temporary intraocular tamponading agent. Chang et al[45] reported a 94% success rate in a series of giant tear repairs, using PFCLs (perfluorotributylamine, perfluorodecalin, and perfluorooctane), and Glaser and associates[85] reported successful retinal reattachment with the use of perfluorooctane. Using PFCLs for giant retinal tears, Le Mer and Kroll reported a 100% reattachment rate.[87]

Kreiger and Lewis[86] used perfluorooctane to manage 11 eyes with giant retinal tears without PVR; this was accomplished without scleral buckling. In all cases they removed the maximum basal vitreous gel and administered endophotocoagulation to the tear edges. C_3F_8 or silicone oil was employed as an intraocular tamponade. Retinal reattachment was accomplished in all eyes, and nine eyes attained final visual acuity of 5/200 or better. Additional necessary major procedures included reoperation for detachment caused by posterior PVR (one eye), removal of silicone oil (four), repeat vitrectomy and membrane removal with photocoagulation (one), cataract extraction (one), removal of a macular pucker (one), postoperative fluid–gas exchanges (four), and anterior chamber tissue plasminogen activator injections for postoperative fibrin reactions (three).

Perfluorocarbon Liquids in PVR

Despite the use of intraocular air, SF_6, perfluorocarbon gas, and silicone oil, it is difficult to tamponade the inferior retina while chorioretinal adhesions are developing after retinal detachment surgery, especially after vitreous traction forms. Furthermore, treatment of giant retinal tears and inferior breaks is difficult with these substances.

Vitreous substitutes with a specific gravity greater than those of infusion fluids offer certain advantages in vitreoretinal surgery. Their high density favors downward movement of the retina, making retinal reattachment easier in many situations, obviating the need for a posterior drainage retinotomy, and facilitating the endolaser application.[88]

The use of PFCL (Fig. 3–10) has changed the surgical management of PVR. Previously, during surgery, anterior PVR was addressed first, followed by dissection of posterior PVR. The use of perfluoroperhydrophenanthrene permits initial dissection of posterior PVR. A three-port pars plana technique is used. Using a pick, an attempt is made to create an edge in the membrane close to the optic nerve head. After initial dissection, a small amount of perfluoroperhydrophenanthrene is injected over the optic nerve, which flattens the adjacent retina. The membrane dissection continues from the posterior to the anterior direction. PFCL facilitates membrane dissection and stabilizes the posterior retina by forcing subretinal fluid out of anteriorly located retinal breaks. Anterior PVR can be dissected and removed subsequently while the posterior retina is attached and kept in place by the weight of the PFCL.[89,90]

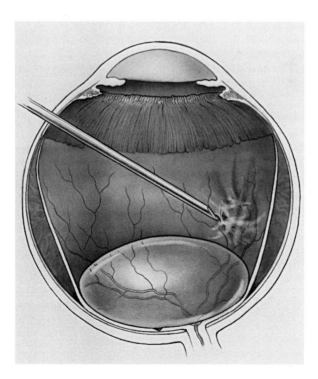

Figure 3–10. Sagittal section showing use of perfluoroperhydrophenanthrene in assisting dissection of preretinal membrane.

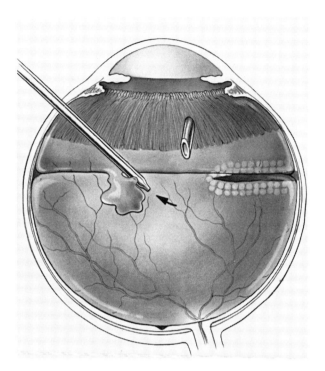

Figure 3–11. Alternative technique of perfluoroperhydrophenanthrene–silicone oil exchange, using special Peyman double-barrel cannula. Silicone is injected through a space between the outer and inner tube while perfluoroperhydrophenanthrene is removed through the open end of the inner tube.

After reattachment of the retina, the PFCL can be exchanged either with gas or silicone oil (Fig. 3–11) to provide a more permanent tamponading effect.[89,90]

Chang and colleagues[44] studied the use of intraoperative PFCLs in the management of PVR. Massive grade D PVR (as classified under the Retina Society system) was present in all 23 eyes; 69.6% (16 eyes) had grade D_3 PVR with closed-funnel configuration. Using PFCLs, retinas were flattened intraoperatively in 21 eyes. This temporary mechanical fixation of the retina expedited epiretinal membrane removal and the release of traction, which was accomplished without the need to perform a posterior retinotomy for internal drainage of subretinal fluid. After a follow-up of 6 months or more, long-term retinal reattachment was found in 65% (15) of eyes.

Carroll et al[89] studied 142 consecutive patients who underwent repair of retinal detachment associated with grades C_2 to D_3 PVR with perfluoroperhydrophenanthrene used as an intraoperative hydrokinetic tool. In nine patients, perfluoroperhydrophenanthrene was also left in the eye for prolonged tamponade. Intraoperative reattachment was obtained in 98% of patient. At final follow-up examination (mean, 7.5 months), 84% of retinas remained attached, and 92% of patients had stable or improved visual acuity. Intraoperative complications included inability to unroll and flatten the retina in three eyes (2%), iatrogenic breaks in three eyes (2%), and sub-retinal hemorrhage in one eye.

PFCL in Management of Dislocated Lenses

In elderly individuals, a dislocated sclerotic nucleus usually can be removed with the vitrectomy instrument only by crushing the nucleus into small pieces and forcing these fragments into the port of the instrument or by the use of phacofragmentation. Both procedures can be protracted and cause retinal injury either because of the lens fragments or because of manipulation of the lens on the retinal surface.

We have successfully used high-density vitreous substitutes such as fluorosilicone oil or perfluoroperhydrophenanthrene to remove dislocated lenses.[91,92] Our operative procedure uses three sclerotomies. A complete vitrectomy is performed, and then the perfluoroperhydrophenanthrene is injected into the vitreous cavity. The dislocated lens floats on the top of the PFCL (Fig. 3–12). The lens is brought into the

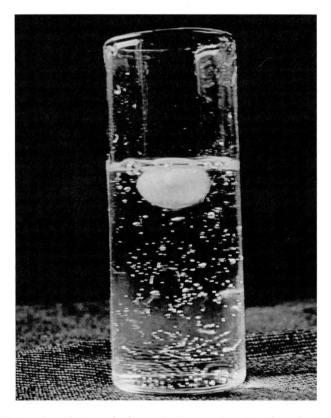

Figure 3–12. In vitro photograph demonstrating a cataractous lens floating on fluorosilicone oil. (From Liu KR, Peyman GA, Chen MS, Chang KB: Use of high-density vitreous substitute in the removal of posteriorly dislocated lenses or intraocular lenses. *Ophthalmic Surg* 1991;22:503–507.)

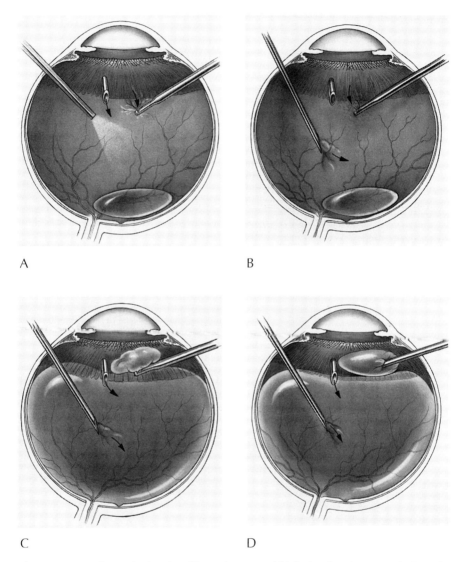

A

B

C

D

Figure 3–13. Schematic drawing illustrating use of high-density vitreous substitute in management of a dislocated lens. **A.** A pars plana vitrectomy is performed. **B.** Perfluoroperhydrophenanthrene is injected to lift up the lens. A lensectomy is performed either with a vitrectomy instrument (**C**) or with a phacofragmentor (**D**). Arrows indicate simultaneous or intermittent infusion of fluid, perfluoroperhydrophenanthrene, or fluorosilicone, as needed. (From Liu KR, Peyman GA, Chen MS, Chang KB: Use of high-density vitreous substitute in the removal of posteriorly dislocated lenses or intraocular lenses. *Ophthalmic Surg* 1991;22:503–507.)

anterior part of the vitreous, where it is removed either with a vitrectomy instrument or a phacofragmentor (Fig. 3–13A–C) combined with a flute needle or aspirating light pipe to stabilize the lens during fragmentation. With the use of PFCL, a hard lens can be brought into the anterior chamber and removed through a corneal incision (Fig. 3–14). No intraoperative complications have been noted.

We successfully removed posteriorly dislocated crystalline lenses or IOLs in a series of 28 patients using perfluoroperhydrophenanthrene in this manner.[92] Korobelnik et al[93] note removal of a posteriorly dislocated lens using a similar technique with a perfluorocarbon liquid. This procedure can be combined with trabeculectomy and insertion of an anterior chamber IOL. After this procedure, control of IOP has been good.

Because of the complexity of lens removal by conventional techniques, posteriorly dislocated lenses have frequently been left in the vitreous until vision-threatening complications occurred. Our method using heavier-than-water vitreous substitutes for lens removal expands the indications for the removal of posteriorly dislocated lenses or IOLs. When fluorosilicone or other PFCLs are used in the management of dislocated lenses or lens fragments, these vitreous substitutes are removed intraoperatively.[91,92,94-100]

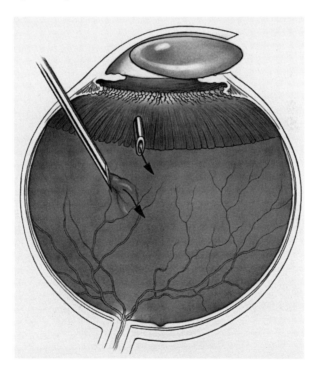

Figure 3–14. Schematic drawing of a dislocated hard (4+ nuclear sclerotic) lens. Perfluoroperhydrophenanthrene is injected, and the dislocated hard lens is elevated and delivered through limbal wound. Arrows indicate simultaneous or intermittent infusion of fluid or fluorosilicone, as needed.

Management of Dislocated Pseudophakos Using Perfluorocarbon Liquid

Several reports document the use of PFCLs to manage posteriorly dislocated intraocular lenses.[91,92,95,99,101] As previously described, PFCLs, with a specific gravity of 1.9 to 2.0, are heavier than water and heavier than a dislocated lens or dislo-

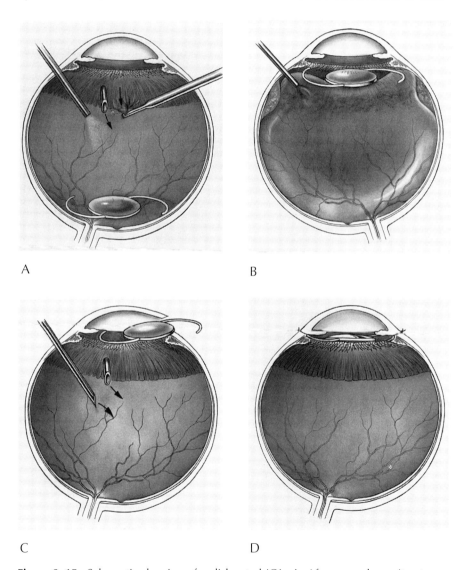

A

B

C

D

Figure 3–15. Schematic drawing of a dislocated IOL. **A.** After pars plana vitrectomy; **B.** perfluoroperhydrophenanthrene is injected and the dislocated IOL is elevated and removed through limbal wound; or **C.** IOL is either removed or **D.** sutured to the ciliary sulcus.

cated pseudophakos. After three sclerotomies are made, a vitrectomy is performed (Fig. 3–15A) and 2 to 3 mL PFCL is injected into the vitreous cavity (Fig. 3–15B). This maneuver lifts the dislocated pseudophakos from the retina, so that it floats on the surface of the PFCL in the vitreous cavity. In case of a dislocated pseudophakos, the haptics can now be grasped easily and removed through a corneal incision or brought through the pars plana and sutured under an already prepared scleral flap (Fig. 3–15C). The use of PFCL protects the retina from accidental injury during surgical manipulation of the IOL in the vitreous cavity. If the pseudophakos accidentally falls back during its retrieval, it will not strike and possibly injure the retina, but will float on the PFCL instead.

Fanous and Friedman[101] described a technique that uses perfluoroperhydrophenanthrene to aid in the transscleral suturing of a posterior chamber IOL to the ciliary sulcus. As PFCL fills the globe, the liquid floats the lens into position behind the pupil. One haptic is grasped with intraocular forceps, and the other is caught in a 10–0 polypropylene loop (Fig. 3–16), which has been threaded through a standard 25-gauge hypodermic needle and inserted into the eye. When the needle is withdrawn, the loop remains inside the eye. The second haptic is similarly secured, and the sutures are tied in the scleral bed, with the haptics stabilized in the ciliary sulcus. Fanous and Friedman[101] found that the use of PFCL facilitates manipulation of dis-

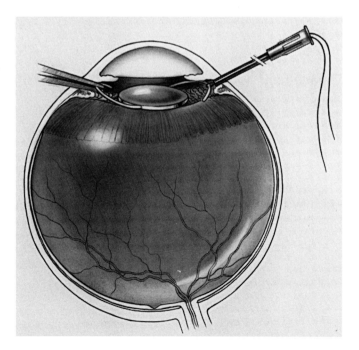

Figure 3–16. Use of perfluoroperhydrophenanthrene in the transscleral suturing of a posterior chamber IOL. The liquid floats the lens into position behind the pupil. One haptic is grasped with intraocular forceps and the other caught in a 10–0 polypropylene loop, which has been threaded through a standard 25-gauge hypodermic needle.

located IOLs and virtually eliminates the risk of damage to the retina from an IOL that sinks back into the vitreous cavity.

In general, we prefer to remove potentially dislocated IOLs and, if needed, replace them with an anterior chamber lens.

Between January 1989 and October 1992, 28 patients were enrolled in the multicenter Vitreon trial.[92] Twelve surgeons at eight participating centers contributed data. Posteriorly dislocated crystalline lenses (n = 20) or IOLs (n = 9, including one patient with both a dislocated crystalline lens and IOL) were successfully removed from all 28 patients with the aid of perfluoroperhydrophenanthrene. PFCL was successfully used as an intraoperative tool to float the crystalline lens or IOL into the midvitreous cavity, thus avoiding dangerous micromanipulation with intraocular instruments in the macular area. When preoperative and postoperative visual acuities were compared, it was found that visual acuity improved in 19 patients (73%), remained unchanged in 4 (15%), and worsened in 3 (12%); two patients were excluded from this calculation because preoperative visual acuity was not known. Final acuity was 20/40 or better in 9 eyes (32%), 20/100 or better in 19 (68%), and 20/400 or better in 24 (86%). Two of the three eyes with decreased acuity lost only one line. Postoperative complications included a recurrent retinal detachment in an eye that suffered from a giant retinal tear and had a posteriorly dislocated crystalline lens following cataract surgery. It was noted in one eye that a droplet of perfluoroperhydrophenanthrene remained in the anterior chamber, but no other ocular complications were found.

Retinal Detachment Associated with Dislocated Crystalline or Intraocular Lenses

Perfluorocarbon liquids have been used as adjuncts to vitrectomy in the management of detached retinas associated with dislocated crystalline or intraocular lenses.[91,92,102,103] While elevating the lens, the PFCL also displaced subretinal fluid through an anterior break in the peripheral detached retina, successfully flattening the retina. The crystalline lens can be removed using previously described techniques followed by endophotocoagulation to the retina surrounding the peripheral retinal tear. An encircling band can then be placed around the peripheral retina.

Lewis and associates,[102] using similar techniques, reported successful treatment of a dislocated crystalline lens and retinal detachment with PFCL in four eyes. The retina was reattached without complication in each eye; after follow-up periods ranging from 6 to 9 months, visual acuity was improved and the retina remained attached in all four eyes.

Massive Suprachoroidal Hemorrhage

The most severe form of choroidal hemorrhage is massive intraoperative suprachoroidal or expulsive hemorrhage. This rare condition occurs when a hemorrhage in the suprachoroidal space is massive enough to result in extrusion of intraocular contents outside the eye or to force the retinal surfaces into near or direct apposition.[104-106] Massive intraoperative choroidal hemorrhage is one of the most severe complications of intraocular surgery; it occurs less commonly after ocular trauma.

Choroidal hemorrhages as a complication of intraocular surgery may occur intraoperatively, in the early postoperative period, or (less commonly) late in the postoperative period.

The incidence of expulsive hemorrhage varies with the type of intraocular surgery. Filtering procedures[107,108] have the highest rate, but the greatest number of incidents of expulsive hemorrhage occur as a result of cataract extraction, because this procedure is so prevalent. The incidence of expulsive hemorrhage after cataract extractions varies from 0.05% to 0.4%.[109] The incidence in most reports is slightly lower in extracapsular procedures than in intracapsular procedures.[110–112] The incidence during or after penetrating keratoplasty has been reported to be 1.08%.[113]

Massive suprachoroidal hemorrhage is a very rare but well-documented complication after scleral buckling procedures.[114,115] Only a few reports mention massive suprachoroidal hemorrhage after pars plana vitrectomy.[104,113]

Different mechanisms have been suggested to explain the pathophysiology of suprachoroidal hemorrhage.[106,116-121] The three mechanisms proposed by Bellows et al[116] include rupture of posterior ciliary arteries or a large vortex vein after either a serous choroidal detachment, hypotony, or trauma. Another mechanism may involve obstruction of venous outflow from the vortex veins caused by compression as a result of either scleral thickening or scleral buckle compression, which raises hydrostatic pressure in the choroidal circulation, resulting in a cascade of events that ends in the formation of a choroidal hemorrhage. Choroidal hemorrhage also may result from direct traumatic laceration of choroidal blood vessels.[106]

Beyer and associates[120] developed an experimental model of expulsive choroidal hemorrhage in rabbits, which may provide new information relating to the cause and prevention of this condition. After sedation with intravenous pentobarbital sodium, rabbits were given lactated Ringer's solution and heparin sodium intravenously. The right eyes were prolapsed, and the central cornea, lens, and anterior vitreous were removed. After surgery, all eyes (100%) developed choroidal effusion, choroidal hemorrhage, or expulsive hemorrhage. The rabbits were killed at various intervals after surgery so that the eyes could be enucleated and processed for light microscopy. After histologically reviewing the eyes, the investigators detected an orderly sequence of events that led to expulsive hemorrhage. This sequence of events is depicted schematically in Fig. 3–17.

Reviews that list predisposing factors of suprachoroidal hemorrhage are not always in agreement. Reported risk factors include old age, glaucoma, aphakic intraocular inflammation, and high myopia.[105] In other studies, patients with cardiovascular disease, high myopia, glaucoma, or aphakia were found to be at greatest risk for developing this complication.[104,122-124]

In one case-controlled epidemiologic study, Speaker and associates[125] identified the following as independent risk factors associated with suprachoroidal hemorrhage: glaucoma, axial length greater than or equal to 25.8 mm, elevated preoperative IOP greater than 18 mm Hg, and a pulse rate greater than or equal to 85 beats

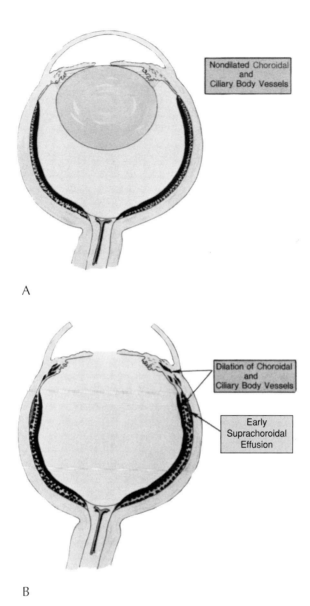

A

B

Figure 3–17. Schematic representation of the sequence of events leading to expulsive hemorrhage. **A.** The normal rabbit eye before cornea and lens removal and anterior vitrectomy. The choroidal and ciliary body vessels are nondilated. **B.** After the cornea, lens, and anterior vitreous are removed, hypotony causes the choroidal and ciliary body vessels to dilate, leading to suprachoroidal effusion. **C.** As the suprachoroidal effusion enlarges, there is stretching and tearing of choroidal vascular attachments, resulting in limited suprachoroidal hemorrhage. **D.** Continued enlargement of the suprachoroidal effusion and hemorrhage leads to ciliary body detachment and tearing of massively dilated ciliary body vessels. **E** (page 170). Presumably, high-pressure bleeding from the torn ciliary body vessels results in expulsive hemorrhage. (From Beyer CF, Peyman GA, Hill JM: Expulsive choroidal hemorrhage in rabbits: A histopathologic study. *Arch Ophthalmol* 1989;107:1648–1653. Copyright 1989, American Medical Association.)

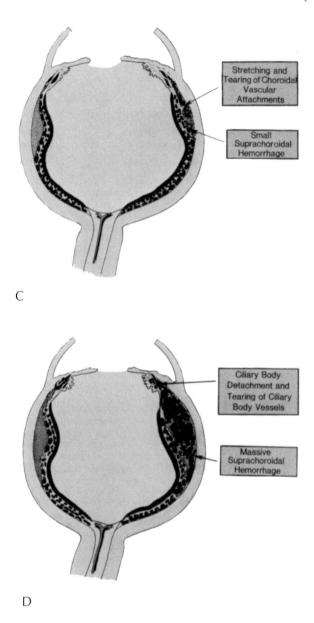

C

D

Figure 3–17 (Continued).

per minute. The contralateral eye of an eye with an expulsive hemorrhage has an increased risk in the future.[111] That risk may be as high as 20%.[112]

Identification of patients at risk for this serious surgical complication is extremely important. Prophylactic treatment of systemic and intraocular risk factors in these individuals is desirable to lessen the possibility of an expulsive hemorrhage

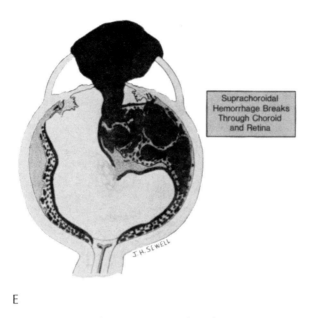

E

Figure 3–17 (Continued).

complicating intraocular surgery. The best opportunity for minimizing the effects of this complication is provided by the use of surgical techniques that allow an immediate tight closure of the globe should an expulsive hemorrhage occur.[125]

Hemorrhagic choroidal detachments occurring at the time of cataract or filtering surgery often may require immediate drainage. Limited choroidal hemorrhages during intraocular surgery may require no treatment and may have a good prognosis.[126] Gressel and colleagues[127] have described delayed nonexpulsive suprachoroidal hemorrhages in patients undergoing filtering surgery in aphakic eyes with glaucoma. Frenkel and Shin,[124] in combining 18 cases of limited delayed suprachoroidal hemorrhages and massive delayed suprachoroidal hemorrhage, have also shown that limited delayed nonexpulsive suprachoroidal hemorrhages occurring postoperatively may not require surgery. However, massive delayed nonexpulsive suprachoroidal hemorrhage usually requires surgical intervention to achieve a favorable visual outcome and to treat postoperative persistent hypotony. Frenkel and Shin[124] suggest that this treatment should include drainage of the suprachoroidal hemorrhage and reformation of the anterior chamber.

Immediate management of expulsive hemorrhage includes watertight wound closure. When performing a rapid closure, the surgeon should avoid damage to the retina from vitreous traction or direct iatrogenic retinal injury. External drainage after wound closure is performed by creating posterior sclerotomies.[128-135]

The use of PFCL to manage suprachoroidal hemorrhages was described by Desai, Peyman, and colleagues (Fig. 3–18).[136] A 360° limbal peritomy was made with two radial relaxing incisions and the rectus muscles tagged using 4–0 silk ties. After the sclera was inspected, 4-mm circumferential sclerotomies were made 5.0 mm posterior to the limbus in three quadrants. A 25-gauge needle was inserted through the inferotemporal limbus in aphakic patients, or through the pars plana into the vitreous cavity, and the needle tip was visualized. Perfluoroperhydrophenanthrene was slowly injected over the retina. As the PFCL moved posteriorly, its tamponading effect forced the suprachoroidal blood to exit through the anterior sclerotomies, aided by gentle pressure on the globe with cotton-tipped applicators. Once the suprachoroidal blood was removed, the inferonasal sclerotomy was closed with 6–0 Vicryl sutures. An inferotemporal sclerotomy was made and a 6-mm infusion cannula secured with 6–0 Vicryl sutures. Next, a pars plana vitrectomy was performed anteriorly, assisted by the operating microscope or by the indirect ophthalmoscope if the cornea was cloudy. After the vitrectomy was complete, perfluoroperhydrophenanthrene was either left in the eye or removed using multiple air–perfluorocarbon exchanges. The sclerotomies were then closed using 6–0 Vicryl sutures. Air or a long-acting gas may be injected through the pars plana in a nonexpansile concentration.

Three patients were treated in this manner, one with a large suprachoroidal detachment with the retina abutting the IOL (Fig. 3–19A). At follow-up 5 months after surgery, complete resolution of the suprachoroidal blood was noted in all patients (Fig. 3–19B). All three had attached retinas and postoperative visual acuities were improved over preoperative visual acuities.

This surgical technique has certain advantages over previously described techniques. Perfluoroperhydrophenanthrene is a heavier-than-water liquid perfluorocarbon with a specific gravity of 2.03.[32] This property allows the liquid perfluorocarbon to flatten the posterior pole when it is injected with the patient in a supine position. The tamponading force is highest in the posterior direction, thereby forcing the suprachoroidal blood anteriorly (Fig. 3–18B). As the blood is pushed anteriorly, it can be removed from an anterior sclerotomy placed 4.0 mm from the limbus. This procedure differs from the technique described by Abrams and associates in 1986,[129] using a continuous-pressure air pump. The sclerotomies were located at the equator. Apparently the posterior location of the sclerotomies was necessary because of the dynamics of air injection. The injection of air, with the patient in a supine position, would cause the major tamponading force to be directed anteriorly (Fig. 3–18C). Because of this, the blood would be forced posteriorly and the sclerotomy would have to be posterior.[129] Desai et al[136] believe their perfluoroperhydrophenanthrene technique allows more complete removal of suprachoroidal blood, with the direction of the tamponading effect reversed from posterior to anterior. The technique of Lakhanpal and associates,[130] in which balanced salt solution is injected into the eye,[130] may provide a more homogeneous tamponading effect than air, but the necessity for posterior sclerotomies as far back as 8 mm suggests that some of the suprachoroidal blood is being forced posteriorly (Fig. 3–18D).

Treatment for massive suprachoroidal hemorrhage has sometimes included vitrectomy.[133,137,138] We used vitrectomy in two of our cases after drainage of the

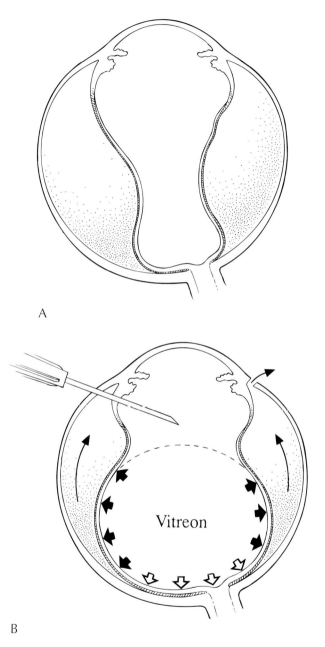

A

B

Figure 3–18. A. Suprachoroidal hemorrhage seen elevating the choroid and retina.
B. The perfluoroperhydrophenanthrene bubble has the greatest tamponading effect
posteriorly. This forces suprachoroidal blood anteriorly and out through the anterior
sclerotomy.

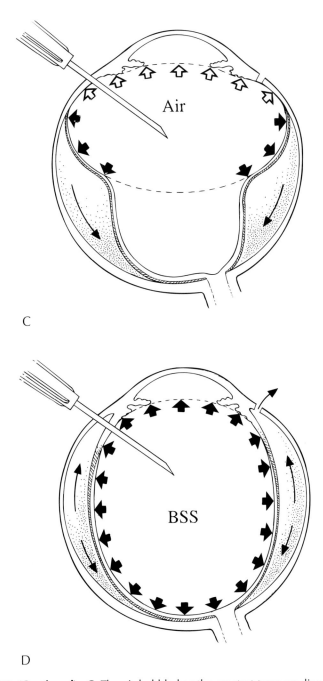

C

D

Figure 3–18 (Continued). C. The air bubble has the greatest tamponading effect anteriorly. This forces the suprachoroidal blood posteriorly. **D.** Balanced salt solution has a more homogeneous tamponading effect. Blood may be moved anteriorly and posteriorly. (Figs. **A**, **C**, and **D** from Desai UR, Peyman GA, Chen CJ, et al: The use of perfluoroperhydrophenanthrene in the management of suprachoroidal hemorrhages. *Ophthalmology* 1992;99:1542–1547. Published courtesy of Opthalmology [1992;99:1542–47.])

suprachoroidal blood. We have found that the high specific gravity of PFCL is beneficial in keeping the retina safely posterior while vitrectomy is performed. The tamponading effect of PFCL pushes the retina and choroid back, and the vitreous is pushed anteriorly where it can be removed with less risk of causing an iatrogenic retinal break.

Another benefit of PFCL is that its injection with simultaneous drainage of suprachoroidal blood allows the eye to maintain a constant force directed toward the posterior pole, with a constant pressure. Fluctuating pressure with hypotony may exacerbate the suprachoroidal hemorrhage.[115,130] The reports by Abrams and associates and Lakhanpal and associates recognized this fact and advocated the importance of maintaining constant pressure in the eye.[129,130]

Another advantage of the use of perfluoroperhydrophenanthrene is that it can be left in the eye, if necessary, for 1 month if subsequent studies prove it to be nontoxic to the retina.[32,33,35] The tamponading effect allows it to keep the retina and choroid flat after the suprachoroidal blood is removed.

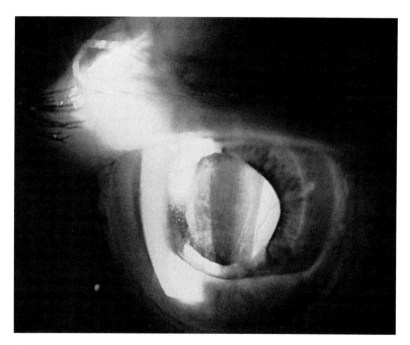

A

Figure 3–19. A. Slit lamp photo of right eye shows retina posterior to the nasal aspect of intraocular lens. **B.** Fundus photo at 5 months follow-up shows the disc and vessels to be within normal limits. (From Desai UR, Peyman GA, Chen CJ, et al: The use of perfluoroperhydrophenanthrene in the management of suprachoroidal hemorrhages. *Ophthalmology* 1992;99:1542–1547. Published courtesy of *Opthalmology* [1992;99:1542–47.])

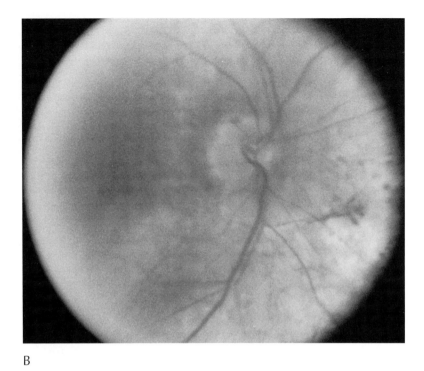

B

Figure 3–19 (Continued).

Perfusion of Perfluorocarbon Liquid in the Management of Traumatic Retinal Detachment with Vitreous Hemorrhage and Anterior Retinal Tear

Traumatic eye injuries are often accompanied by vitreous hemorrhage and retinal detachment caused by peripheral tears (Fig. 3–20A–D). After the diagnosis is established by the use of ultrasound, the surgeon must decide when to intervene surgically. Because of the inadequate visualization of the fundus, he or she must also decide the best approach to prevent retinal injury.

After initial wound repair and prophylaxis of endophthalmitis, we wait 1 week, during which time the posterior hyaloid separates from the retina,[140] providing a space for dissection of the opaque vitreous from the detached retina. Three standard sclerotomies are performed. The site of the infusion cannula is positioned more toward the pars plicata. Using the endoilluminator and a vitrectomy instrument, the surgeon initiates an anterior vitrectomy and lensectomy if the lens has been damaged. The amount of suction and infusion should be kept to the minimum to avoid ballooning of the already detached retina. As soon as the surgeon cuts the detached posterior hyaloid, the vitrectomy instrument is removed and a 20-gauge blunt needle connected to a syringe with 5 mL PFCL is inserted in the vitreous cavity. The tip of

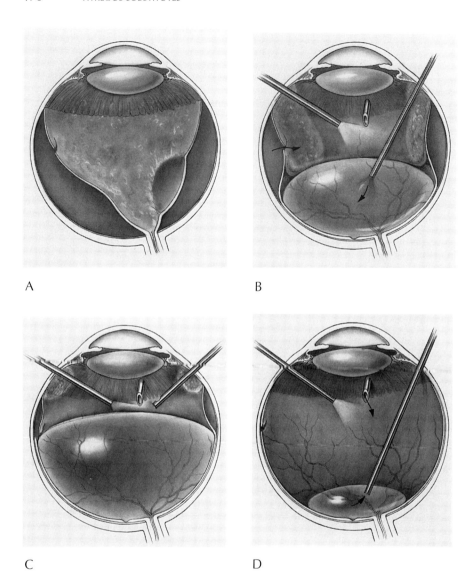

A

B

C

D

Figure 3–20. A. Graphic depiction of traumatic retinal detachment with vitreous hemorrhage. **B.** Using the endoilluminator and a vitrectomy instrument, the surgeon performs anterior vitrectomy and cuts through the posterior hyaloid membrane. **C.** Perfluoroperhydrophenanthrene is injected into the retrohyaloid space. It fills the posterior part of the vitreous and flattens the posterior retina while the subretinal fluid is pressed out from the anteriorly located retinal hole or tear. Perfluoroperhydrophenanthrene separates the posterior hyaloid membrane from the retina and pushes the vitreous hemorrhage anteriorly. **D.** Vitrectomy is completed in the anterior part of the vitreous, removing most of the vitreous opacities. Perfluoroperhydrophenanthrene is removed by air–perfluoroperhydrophenanthrene exchange.

the needle is passed through the opening in the posterior hyaloid membrane in the retrohyaloid space. PFCL is injected gradually (Fig. 1–20B) into the space between the posterior hyaloid membrane and the detached retina. The height of the infusion bottle is lowered as the vitreous cavity gradually fills with PFCL. As the PFCL fills the posterior part of the vitreous and flattens the posterior retina (Fig. 3–20C), the subretinal fluid is pressed out from the anteriorly located (still invisible) retinal hole or tears. During this procedure, the entire vitreous containing the hemorrhage is pushed forward toward the anterior part of the vitreous cavity. At this stage, the vitrectomy instrument is reinserted into the vitreous cavity and vitrectomy is performed in the anterior part of the vitreous until the majority of the vitreous opacities are removed. More PFCL can be injected to facilitate dissection of the posterior hyaloid membrane and to flatten the retinal periphery. The vitrectomy is completed and the retina is inspected for retinal holes, tears, or disinsertions. Often a schlieren is seen at the site of retinal holes as the subretinal fluid exits toward the vitreous cavity, which indicates the site of a retinal defect.

Endolaser or cryotherapy is applied to the retinal hole. Perfluoroperhy-drophenanthrene may be left inside the eye if the anterior lens capsule has been preserved during surgery; otherwise, it can be removed by air–perfluoroper-hydrophenanthrene (Fig. 3–20D) or perfluoroperhydrophenanthrene–silicone exchange. The operation concludes with further endolaser application to the peripheral retina, and suturing of an encircling band to the sclera to support the anterior retina.

Retinal Detachment Associated with Choroidal Coloboma

Choroidal colobomas are rare congenital abnormalities consisting of hypoplastic retina overlying an area without RPE and choroid.[141-144] This ocular defect, caused by dysembryogenesis of the fetal fissure, is associated with retinal detachment in approximately 23% to 42% of eyes.[142,144-146] These retinal detachments, which frequently occur in younger individuals, constitute 0.5% of all juvenile retinal detachments.[143,147]

Poor anatomic success rates ranging from 35% to 57% have been reported in previous studies, in which scleral buckling has been used to treat retinal detachments associated with choroidal colobomas.[148-151] Scleral buckling in eyes with retinal detachment associated with choroidal colobomas is only indicated in individuals with peripheral retinal breaks.[142]

In 1983, Gonvers[151] reported the successful treatment of a retinal detachment in an eye with a choroidal coloboma using vitrectomy, silicone oil injection, and laser photocoagulation. Hanneken and associates[142] reported the results of vitreous surgery in eight eyes with large posterior colobomas associated with retinal detachments characterized either by posterior holes or by a rhegmatogenous appearance and lack of evidence of peripheral retinal breaks. Eyes with optic nerve pit, morning glory syndrome, or isolated optic nerve coloboma were excluded from this series.

An axial vitrectomy followed lensectomy in all eyes. Separation of the posterior hyaloid from the retina was required to prevent recurrent retinal detachment from later postoperative vitreous contraction. Most eyes demonstrated almost complete attachment of the posterior cortex to the retina. Attempts to release all vitreoretinal traction by removing the posterior hyaloid membranes from the retinal surface as far peripherally as the vitreous base were difficult in some eyes as a result of the extent of vitreoretinal adherence, especially in areas of detached retina. This strong adhesion between the vitreous and retina was usually a result of the young age of the patient. An encircling scleral buckle was placed when retinal attachment could not be achieved or when iatrogenic peripheral retinal tears were created.

Retinal breaks, which are often slitlike, can be difficult to identify in the absence of normal underlying RPE and choroid.[142] To identify breaks in the base of the coloboma, the investigators looked for schlieren phenomenon while applying minimal aspiration above the coloboma.

Hanneken and associates found a single retinal break in four eyes and two retinal breaks in an additional eye.[142] Cyanoacrylate retinopexy was used to close and seal the breaks after an air–fluid exchange and endodrainage, which removed all subretinal fluid in the coloboma. This drainage was accomplished through preexisting retinal holes or retinotomies. Creation of an adequate chorioretinal adhesion surrounding the retinal breaks using photocoagulation or cryopexy is impossible because of underlying depigmented tissues. Endocryotherapy or endolaser photocoagulation then was applied to normal retina at the site of the coloboma to create a chorioretinal adhesion, preventing extrusion of any recurrent subretinal fluid that reaccumulated in the base of the coloboma.

An intraocular tamponade was achieved with SF_6, C_3F_8, or silicone oil.

The authors reported anatomic success in seven of the eight eyes, while the number of surgical procedures ranged from one to five per eye. The most frequent complication was PVR.

McDonald et al[143] were successful in reattaching the retina after vitreous surgery in seven eyes with retinal breaks within or at the margin of a choroidal coloboma. When possible, a standard three-port pars plana vitrectomy was performed under general anesthesia, as retrobulbar injection carried a high risk of penetrating the ectatic sclera found in these eyes. The surgical technique combined vitrectomy, membrane peeling, endodrainage, and air–fluid exchange through preexisting retinal breaks or retinotomies, and endophotocoagulation to part or all of the rim of the choroidal coloboma. Vision improved in all but two eyes. Both eyes had choroidal colobomas involving the optic nerve. The investigators proposed peripapillary endophotocoagulation involving the papillomacular bundle in these eyes. To prevent damage to the papillomacular bundle, they used postoperative krypton laser.

Gopal et al[152] described the management of retinal detachment secondary to retinal breaks in coloboma areas in 17 eyes. Treatment consisted of vitrectomy followed by simultaneous drainage of subretinal fluid through the retinal tear in the coloboma area during air–fluid exchange in 12 eyes and through a preexisting or accidental peripheral retinal tear in the remaining five eyes.

The investigators noted that eyes are difficult to seal with retinopexy alone in the absence of choroid and RPE. Three rows of endophotocoagulation were applied along the entire margin of the coloboma. In some cases, cryopexy was applied along the extreme anterior margin of the coloboma to ensure formation of a chorioretinal seal around the complete margin of the coloboma. The authors advocated postoperative krypton laser treatment to the functional area of the disc margin when the coloboma involves the optic nerve, to avoid destroying the papillomacular bundle nerve fiber layer.[153]

Silicone oil was used as a temporary internal tamponade. It provided a prolonged tamponade not possible with a gas bubble while an adequate chorioretinal adhesion formed. Additionally, silicone oil was able to tamponade the entire coloboma for the period required, which would have been difficult or impossible if gas had been used.

A 100% reattachment rate was present at 2 months, but a 33% recurrence rate followed silicone oil removal.

When a retinal break is located inferiorly, as in retinal detachment associated with coloboma, the ability of gas or silicone oil to tamponade the break is compromised. Treatment often requires difficult positioning, induces lens changes, and makes posterior pole view difficult for necessary postoperative laser photocoagulation.

Lee and colleagues[154] reported a case in which a recurrent retinal detachment associated with coloboma after vitreous surgery and SF_6 gas injection was successfully repaired in outpatient surgery using perfluoroperhydrophenanthrene and endolaser photocoagulation. The patient had previously undergone a penetrating keratoplasty for pseudophakic bullous keratopathy in the affected eye and had visual acuity of count fingers at 2 feet. The anterior segment examination showed clear corneal graft. Fundus examination showed a total bullous retinal detachment, including the macula and a 3–disc-diameter-size choroidal coloboma inferonasal to the disc. The detachment involved the margin of the coloboma. No retinal break was seen preoperatively in the area of the coloboma or in the periphery. The patient subsequently underwent a repair of the retinal detachment. Intraoperatively, two small operculated peripheral retinal breaks, thought to be responsible for the detachment, were found at the 12 o'clock and 7 o'clock meridians.

A three-port pars plana vitrectomy was performed and the retina reattached. During follow-up examination 2 days later, however, subretinal fluid had reaccumulated in the inferonasal retina involving the area of coloboma. The recurrent subretinal fluid was thought to originate from continuous leakage through a probable retinal defect in the coloboma. The patient was taken to an outpatient surgical suite, where topical anesthesia was administered. Two milliliters perfluoroperhydrophenanthrene was injected through the pars plana, and an equal amount of air was removed. No special positioning of the patient's head after the perfluoroperhydrophenanthrene injection was required because the retinal defect was located inferiorly. However, the patient was advised to keep her head slightly elevated when lying down. Several days after the perfluoroperhydrophenanthrene injection, when the retina was completely flat, argon laser photocoagulation was performed around the coloboma and over the buckle. Perfluoroperhydrophenanthrene was removed 4 weeks later in an operating room on an outpatient basis using pars plana air–fluid exchange. At 7 months' follow-up, the retina remained flat. The patient's visual acuity was counting fingers at 5 feet. The poor vision was thought to be attributable to cystoid macular edema and changes in the corneal graft.

Lee et al[154] concluded that in this case perfluoroperhydrophenanthrene provided a convenient tool to reattach the retina. It provided the longstanding inferior retinal flattening needed for development of a strong chorioretinal scar after photocoagulation.

PFCL in Management of Retinal Detachment Following Prosthokeratoplasty

Prosthokeratoplasty is a procedure in which the cornea is permanently replaced with an artificial keratoprosthesis. It is used in patients with bilateral disabling corneal blindness when penetrating keratoplasty is likely to fail.[155,156] Despite excellent initial visual results, there can be many long-term complications: retinal detachment, endophthalmitis, uveitis, leakage around or extrusion of the keratoprosthesis, and epithelial down-growth.[155-162]

Retinal detachment occurs in up to 20% of keratoprosthetic cases.[155,159,162] Prosthokeratoplasty involves cataract extraction, iridectomy, and vitrectomy. Vitrectomy must usually be done with an open sky technique because visualization is poor through the scarred cornea. A complete vitrectomy cannot be accomplished with this technique, and the remaining vitreous may contract and cause a retinal detachment. Although successful repair using a 360° wide buckle has been reported, limited fundus visualization (less than 30°) and failure to address the associated vitreous pathology often result in failure.

Paris, Peyman, and colleagues[34] reported the successful treatment of rhegmatogenous retinal detachment after Cardona prosthokeratoplasty with a surgical technique that included pars plana vitrectomy, endolaser photocoagulation, peripheral cryopexy, scleral buckling, and the use of perfluoroperhydrophenanthrene to achieve and maintain attachment (Figs. 3–21, 3–22). This PFCL was allowed to remain in the eye for 3 weeks after the operation. Postoperative visual acuity stabilized at functional levels, and no ocular complications, adverse reactions, or redetachment were observed.

After induction of general anesthesia, the patient was prepared and draped as for vitreous surgery. Because implantation of the keratoprosthesis device required periosteal grafting and permanent tarsorrhaphy with excision of tarsal plates, skin incisions became necessary. The first incision was made medially and laterally in the superior sulcus and extended to points above the canthal tendons. A similar incision was made in the inferior sulcus. To preclude possible central lid ischemia, care was taken to avoid disruption of blood supply at the canthal borders. The superior and inferior rectus muscles were isolated and harnessed with 3–0 silk sutures. The dissection was complete when bare sclera was exposed.

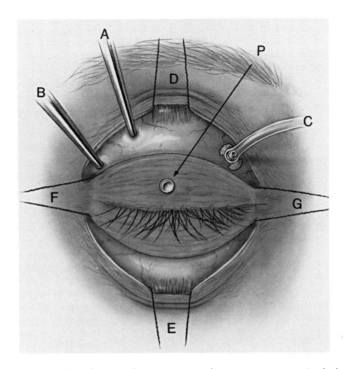

Figure 3–21. Surgical technique for managing rhegmatogenous retinal detachment after prosthokeratoplasty. Skin incisions, placement of sclerotomies, and instrumentation before vitrectomy: (A) endoilluminator; (B) vitrectomy probe; (C) infusion cannula; (D,E) isolated recti muscles; (F,G) isolated canthal tendons; (P) keratoprosthetic device.

Hemostasis was achieved with cauterization. A sclerotomy was placed in the superonasal quadrant 4.0 mm lateral and 2.0 mm anterior to the superior rectus muscle, thus ensuring entry through the pars plana. A 6.0-mm infusion cannula was inserted through the sclerotomy and anchored to the globe with a 6–0 Vicryl suture. Two similar sclerotomies were placed in the superotemporal quadrant. The endoilluminator was placed through the more inferior sclerotomy and held by the assistant. A permanent endoilluminator was sutured to the sclera. The vitrectomy probe was inserted through the more superior sclerotomy, and a pars plana vitrectomy was performed under direct visualization through the keratoprosthesis using an indirect ophthalmoscope with its illumination turned off. This technique eliminated unwanted light reflexes produced with an external illuminating source.

Perfluoroperhydrophenanthrene was injected over the posterior pole, causing the hydraulic displacement of subretinal fluid through the peripheral retinal break and reattachment of the retina (Fig. 3–22B). If the hole was located posterior to the ora serrata, the partial air–fluid exchange would prevent anterior trapping of subretinal fluid, permitting complete drainage of subretinal fluid. Endolaser photocoag-

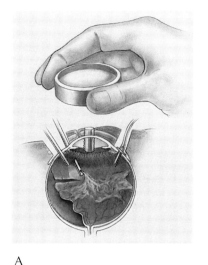

A

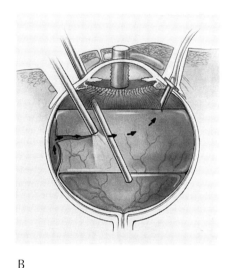

B

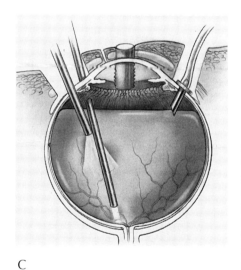

C

Figure 3–22. A. Pars plana vitrectomy with visualization through indirect ophthalmoscopy. **B.** Partial air–fluid exchange followed by perfluoroperhydrophenanthrene injection. Fluid is hydraulically displaced from the subretinal space through the peripheral retinal break. **C.** An endolaser photocoagulation is performed.

ulation was applied prophylactically, encircling the posterior pole (Fig. 3–22C). The endoilluminator and vitrectomy probe were removed from the eye, and the sclerotomies were closed with 6–0 Vicryl sutures.

Because the location of the retinal break could not be visualized, 360° peripheral retinal cryopexy was applied. A no. 20 encircling element was passed around the globe and secured in each quadrant with 5–0 Dacron, partial-thickness mattress sutures. The infusion cannula was clamped and removed, and the sclerotomy was closed with a 6–0 Vicryl suture. The rectus muscle traction sutures were removed, and subcutaneous tissues were closed with a 6–0 Vicryl suture. The overlying skin was reapproximated with 6–0 silk suture. Postoperative prone positioning was not needed because the high specific gravity of perfluoroperhydrophenanthrene provided a posterior tamponading effect.

Three weeks postoperatively, the patient returned to surgery, at which time the perfluoroperhydrophenanthrene was removed to avoid possible retinal toxicity and emulsification. Perfluoroperhydrophenanthrene was removed passively through a 20-gauge flute needle under balanced saline irrigation. Sequential air–fluid exchanges were performed to ensure complete removal. The operative technique was similar to the initial procedure. Visualization was accomplished by indirect ophthalmoscopy, whereas endoillumination, infusion, and the air–fluid exchange were performed through separate sclerotomies. The retina was inspected at the conclusion of surgery.

Perfluoroperhydrophenanthrene has sufficient density to displace subretinal fluid anteriorly, allowing it to exit through peripheral retinal breaks.

The Use of Perfluorocarbon Liquid in Surgical Management of Retinopathy of Prematurity

Management of stage 5 retinopathy of prematurity (ROP) is complicated by many factors. Among these are the small size of the eye, inability to dilate the pupils, lack of pars plana, circular contraction of the anterior part of the vitreous, forming a fibrous membrane behind the lens capsule, and an attached posterior hyaloid, which cannot be peeled off from the surface of the retina. Factors that work in the surgeon's favor in these complex circumstances are the occupation of a large area behind the iris by the lens and the extent of retinal detachment—specifically, the absence of a closed funnel (Fig. 3–23).

In our experience, as with Maguire and Trese,[163] the use of an infusion cannula inserted either through the anterior chamber or pars plicata is often too traumatic for these small eyes. An anterior chamber cannula is also unsatisfactory because it can move and is often in the way of the surgeon's view. Our approach involves the use of two sclerotomies performed just behind the iris root. The first is generally made at the 3 o'clock position for the left eye and 2:30 for the right. Using a sharp microvitreoretinal (MVR) blade, the surgeon enters the lens with the blade through an area located a distance of 0.5 mm behind the iris root. The sclerotomy is enlarged with the same MVR blade to 1.5 times its original size to accommodate an infusion light pipe easily without dislodging the collagenous fibers and vitreous condensation at the vitreous base. These internal structures have to be cut carefully with a sharp blade; otherwise, the ciliary body will be detached during the entry of the infusion light pipe. As soon as the infusion cannula enters the lens, the infusion is started, and the lens is hydrated.

At this point, using the MVR blade, the surgeon creates a second sclerotomy; this is generally located 140° in the opposite field of the initial sclerotomy, but can be modified depending on which structures the surgeon desires to approach with ease

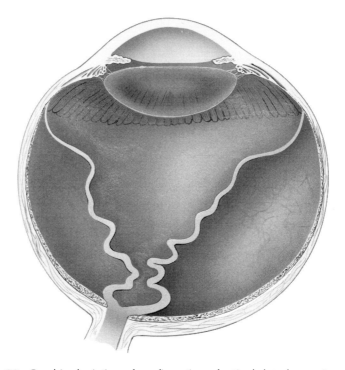

Figure 3–23. Graphic depiction of configuration of retinal detachment in retinopathy of prematurity, showing detached retina with anterior open funnel.

after the lensectomy is completed. The internal structure of the second sclerotomy is cut to achieve a size of at least 1.5 times the length normally needed for insertion of a 20-gauge vitrectomy instrument. As soon as the MVR blade is removed, the vitrectomy instrument is inserted in the lens. Using the infusion light pipe and the vitrectomy instruments, the lens cortex and nucleus are mixed and gradually aspirated until the entire cortex is removed intracapsularly (Fig. 3–24A-B).

If the retinal detachment has an open funnel, the surgeon can now cut the posterior capsule and a part of vitreous condensation located behind the lens capsule, using the vitrectomy instrument. It is, however, not unusual to have difficulty engaging the lens capsule or the condensed vitreous with the vitrectomy instrument. For this reason, the vitrectomy instrument is removed and incising is performed with vitreous scissors. Then, using a 23-gauge needle on a syringe containing 2 mL perfluoroperhydrophenanthrene, the surgeon enters the vitreous cavity through the space created by the lensectomy. After the needle reaches the midvitreous, the surgeon injects PFCL on the surface of the retina. The infusion fluid and the liquid part of the vitreous are displaced anteriorly and exit through the previously prepared large sclerotomy.

With the injection of perfluoroperhydrophenanthrene, the posterior part of the retina flattens to the extent allowed by retinal contractions caused by retinal folds or

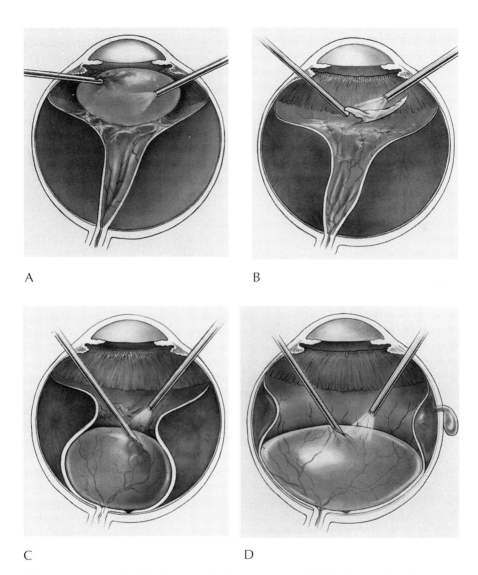

A

B

C

D

Figure 3–24. Use of PFCL in the surgical management of ROP. **A.** Insertion of vitrectomy instrument and infusion light pipe in the lens. **B.** Lensectomy using infusion light pipe and vitrectomy instrument. **C.** Injection of perfluoroperhydrophenanthrene to reattach posterior retina. **D.** Anterior drainage of subretinal fluid prior to placement of encircling no. 40 band to support peripheral retina.

by persistent vitreous adhesions to the optic disc (Fig. 3–24C). If the retinal detachment has a closed configuration, the surgeon uses vitreous scissors to cut the posterior capsule and the anterior part of the vitreous fibers to gain access to the midvitreous cavity. Then using the previously described maneuver, the surgeon injects PFCL toward the posterior pole through the space created by the scissors. After PFCL injection, the posterior retina tends to reattach while the anterior retina is still detached and adherent to the fibrous tissue composed of vitreous base and posterior lens capsule. The surgeon then uses angulated vitreous scissors to cut radially the more distinctly visible anterior contraction of the vitreous base.

At this stage, one can see the anteriorly contracted retina with neovascular tissue extending into the pars plana or plicata. Radial incisions created by scissors are made under high magnification, avoiding the retina and neovascular tissue. As soon as a generous opening is created, the scissors are removed. If needed, additional PFCL is injected inside the eye. Because of its density, PFCL can maintain the shape of the eye, even if the infusion light pipe is removed. Further flattening of the retina may be achieved by injection of perfluoroperhydrophenanthrene and simultaneous drainage of subretinal fluid (Fig. 3–24D). If the surgeon has achieved considerable flattening of the retina during surgery, the PFCL should be exchanged for either gas or silicone injected inside the eye. The anterior lens capsule is removed to prevent subsequent opacification. The sclerotomies are closed, and a no. 40 band is passed under the previously prepared U-shaped 5–0 Dacron sutures located just anterior to the equator of the globe. A moderate buckle is produced by tightening the encircling band. If the IOP is high, some fluid or gas can be removed through the sclerotomies from the posterior chamber. The anterior retina with the neovascular tissue located anterior to the buckle is now coagulated with a single row of cryocoagulation. Dexamethasone (400 μg) is injected inside the eye, and the conjunctiva is closed.

PFCL for Subretinal Surgery

Lambert et al[164] have used PFCLs during the excision of subfoveal membranes to control hemorrhagic complications. After removal of the subretinal neovascular membrane, a bubble of PFCL injected through an infusion light pipe tamponaded any bleeding from the subretinal space while flattening the retina and allowing endophotocoagulation to be applied to the retinotomy site. Near the end of the procedure, the perfluorocarbon was removed during an air–fluid exchange.

PFCL in Diabetic Retinal Detachment

Perfluorocarbons are used in combined traction rhegmatogenous diabetic retinal detachment or when an iatrogenic retinal tear is created during dissection of fibrovascular tissue.[165,166] Usually an encircling band is placed before vitrectomy. Initially, a central and peripheral vitrectomy is performed, relieving anterior–posterior traction. Membranes then are removed. An attempt is made to remove the membrane in one piece to avoid segmentation. Because blood tends to stick to the retina, making complete removal difficult, it is removed immediately after diathermy of bleeding vessels. In cases in which intravitreal silicone will be needed, all residual fibrotic tissue is removed to minimize reproliferation. The retina must be cleaned well, removing all blood and cellular debris. The vitrectomy must always include removal of vitreous in the area of the vitreous base to prevent later retrolenticular proliferation by removing the scaffold for this fibrovascular ingrowth.

Better flattening and anatomic apposition of the retina against the underlying RPE are provided by the use of PFCL, which displaces subretinal fluid in a posterior-to-anterior direction, than by using air–fluid or silicone–fluid exchanges where the tamponading agent fills the eye in an anterior-to-posterior direction. These factors facilitate laser photocoagulation with the endolaser or indirect ophthalmoscope delivery systems. The optics of the eye filled with perfluorocarbon, in contrast to oil, are excellent for endophotocoagulation, which may be performed with standard laser. After laser treatment, perfluorocarbon–gas or perfluorocarbon–saline exchange is performed.

PFCL in Endophthalmitis

Forlini et al[167] have described the use of PFCL in the surgical management of endophthalmitis. In a progressed stage, the vitreous cavity is filled with a very dense, purulent mass. These masses are frequently opaque and adherent to the internal limiting membrane of the retina.

Because orientation inside the vitreous cavity may be difficult, the retina may inadvertently be cut, or iatrogenic tears may be created during manipulation of membranes adherent to the retina. Vitrectomy starts centrally and proceeds toward the periphery. As surgery progresses, PFCL is injected to create a central bubble. The enlarging bubble assists in removal of membranes by balancing traction on the membranes. After vitrectomy in an eye with endophthalmitis (not including the posterior pole), PFCL can be injected so a bubble covers the posterior pole. Then intravitreal antibiotics are injected with the bubble protecting the macula from contact with the antimicrobial agent and possible toxicity. After a predetermined period, the antibiotic is washed out of the vitreous cavity, the PFCL bubble removed, and gas, fluid, or silicone oil is injected into the vitreous cavity.

PFCL in Retinal Incarceration

Retinal incarceration in the sclerotomy site is a serious complication. Withdrawal of the vitrectomy instrument in an eye with an elevated IOP can cause rapid egress of intraocular fluid, which carries forward the detached retina. Treatment may involve disengaging the retina from the sclerotomy lips and repositioning it inside the eye with a blunt-tipped instrument, followed by an air–fluid exchange. Cryocoagulation and a scleral buckling procedure should be performed in these cases.

An open sclerotomy, associated with increased IOP produced by a high flow rate of infusion fluid, predisposes to retinal incarceration. Untreated, this condition creates stiff retinal folds, which cannot settle on the peripheral scleral buckle.

The usual method of management is excision of the extruded vitreous and blunt repositioning of the retina, combined with an air–fluid exchange to flatten the

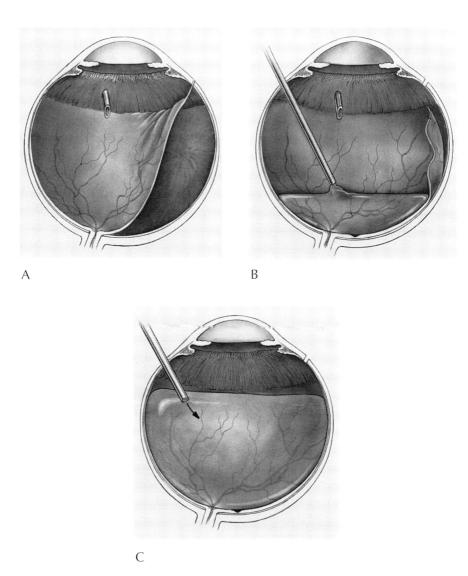

Figure 3–25. Management of retina incarcerated in the sclerotomy. **A.** Schematic drawing of retinal incarceration in a pars plana sclerotomy. **B.** Intravitreal injection of perfluoroperhydrophenanthrene pulls the retina back in the vitreous cavity. **C.** Further injection of the perfluoroperhydrophenanthrene flattens the peripheral retina.

peripheral retina.[153] This technique forces the subretinal fluid posteriorly, and because of incomplete separation of the retina from the incarceration site, results in retinal distortion and permanent retinal fold. To treat an incarcerated retina, Peyman and colleagues[168] developed a surgical technique using perfluoroperhydrophenanthrene.

After retinal incarceration is diagnosed (Fig. 3–25A), the infusion bottle is lowered to the level of the patient's head, reducing IOP. Perfluoroperhydrophenanthrene is injected with a 25-gauge needle on a 5-cc syringe through a separate sclerotomy in the midvitreous cavity (Fig. 3–25B). The high specific gravity of this vitreous substitute causes retraction of the incarcerated retina and forces the subretinal fluid anteriorly (Fig. 3–25C). As the PFCL fills up the vitreous cavity, the detached retina is flattened in the posterior-to-anterior direction. Further vitrectomy may be performed as needed while perfluoroperhydrophenanthrene stabilizes the posterior retina. The fundus is examined by indirect ophthalmoscopy to ensure that the retina is properly released from the sclerotomy site and, if needed, additional vitrectomy is performed to cut the remaining traction. Endophotocoagulation of the peripheral retina, combined with an encircling element, may be employed to prevent a retinal detachment in the postoperative period. At the end of surgery, perfluoroperhydrophenanthrene can be replaced with gas or silicone oil through the infusion cannula.

Management of Subretinal Perfluorocarbon Liquid

Removal of subretinal PFCL from the subretinal space (Fig. 3–26A–B) requires a posterior retinotomy. Infusion of irrigating solution through the infusion cannula is performed simultaneously with removal of the PFCL through an extrusion needle

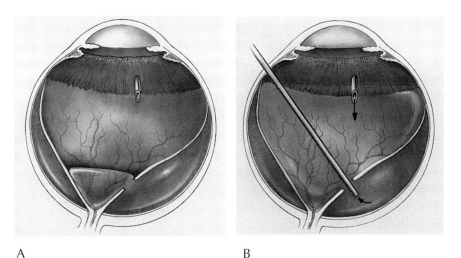

A   B

Figure 3–26. Management of subretinal PFCL. **A.** Graphic representation of PFCL under the retina. **B.** Posterior retinotomy is performed. Infusion fluid enters the eye through a cannula while PFCL is aspirated through an extrusion needle from the subretinal space.

inserted through the retinotomy, until complete removal of the PFCL is achieved. After complete removal of foreign substances from the subretinal space, the retinotomies are coagulated with endolaser. The retina then can be tamponaded with appropriate vitreous substitutes.[164]

Control of Bleeding During Pars Plana Vitrectomy

Skolik et al[169] investigated the use of liquid perfluorocarbon as an adjunct to control bleeding resistant to conventional techniques during pars plana vitrectomy in 20 eyes (17 diabetic, 3 traumatic). The investigators defined bleeding as uncontrolled where the source could not be identified or it occurred from two or more sites that could not be stopped by conventional techniques, including IOP elevation, air–fluid exchange, or bipolar diathermy. Uncontrolled bleeding complicates surgery by impairing visualization and prolonging surgical time.

During pars plana vitrectomy, a sufficient amount of either perfluorooctane or perfluorodecalin was slowly injected over the optic nerve until the source of the uncontrolled bleeding was covered. A volume sufficient to cover the arcades in eyes with proliferative diabetic retinopathy was usually sufficient, whereas in eyes with trauma, a complete fill was needed to stop the bleeding. Intraocular injection of the PFCLs stopped the uncontrolled bleeding in all eyes. In many eyes, the PFCL forced the blood outward from the posterior pole, which increased surgical field visibility while facilitating safe removal of the blood by aspiration. Additional recurrent intraoperative bleeding was not observed.

Animal experiments were performed to determine the mechanism by which the PFCL stopped intraocular bleeding.[169] A hemostatic effect could not be demonstrated. The investigators suggested that PFCL sequesters the clot at the site of bleeding, which controls intraocular hemorrhage.

Removal of Intraocular Foreign Bodies

Experimental studies by Resnick and associates[170] simulated a human eye with a foreign body in the vitreous cavity. The investigators placed several commonly encountered foreign bodies, including wire, glass, gravel, and cilia, in a vessel to which both water and perfluorooctane were added. These foreign bodies floated to the interface between both liquids. Based on these results, the authors suggest that PFCL may assist in the removal of foreign bodies. This heavy liquid, when used as an instrument to elevate foreign bodies in the vitreous cavity, may avoid potential retinal complications during the intraocular manipulation required to retrieve some foreign bodies from the vitreous cavity or retinal surface. Additionally, the high specific gravity allows the PFCL to act as a cushion, which, by supporting the foreign body, prevents damage from the foreign body accidentally falling back on the retina. In the presence of a concurrent retinal detachment, these heavy liquids may flatten the retina while the foreign body is being removed.[170]

Perfluorocarbons in the Treatment of Retinal Ischemia

Perfluorotributylamine, with oxygen solubility 13 times greater than the vitreous,[171] was evaluated as a potential oxygen reservoir with a possible therapeutic function in treating retinal ischemia. Fluorine-19 nuclear magnetic resonance spectroscopy (^{19}F NMR) was used to evaluate the oxygen flux in rabbit eyes filled with the vitreous substitute perfluorotributylamine. Studies demonstrated the rate of increase in perfluorotributylamine PO_2 was 2.34 ± 0.67 mm Hg/min in rabbits breathing 95% O_2 and 5% CO_2. After cessation of ventilation with high levels of oxygen and return to room air, the blood PO_2 returned in 5 minutes to a constant level, whereas the time constant for clearance of O_2 from perfluorotributylamine in vitrectomized eyes was 59.8 ± 9.6 minutes.

After preoxygenation of perfluorotributylamine with 100% oxygen, which increased the PO_2 above 150 mm Hg immediately before injecting the vitreous substitute into the vitreous cavity, the time constant of O_2 clearance was 69.6 ± 12.6 minutes.[172]

Both studies[171,172] demonstrated that when perfluorotributylamine is used as an oxygen reservoir after oxygenation or perfluorotributylamine in the vitreous cavity, PO_2 levels decrease over approximately a 1-hour period. The time during which perfluorotributylamine could act as an oxygen reservoir might be increased in terms of hours by fully oxygenating the perfluorocarbon to 760 mm Hg. The investigators[172] concluded that further studies must be completed to determine if perfluorotributylamine placed in the vitreous cavity could be efficacious in temporarily maintaining retinal function in a hypoxic eye such as might be found in branch retinal vein occlusion, diabetic retinopathy, and retinal vascular insufficiency, which produce areas of inner retinal ischemia.

In separate animal experiments, Wilson and associates[173] demonstrated that oxygenated perfluorocarbons can increase retinal tolerance to ischemia by supplying oxygen to ischemic retina. The oxygenated perfluorocarbon fluid met some but not all of the metabolic requirements of the ischemia retina. The investigators note that this property may be useful in eyes in which IOP elevation during surgery to prevent bleeding results in an ischemic retina. Oxygenated perfluorocarbons may also in the future facilitate the transport and redistribution of intravitreal oxygen in ocular diseases associated with focal retinal ischemia.

Additional Indications for PFCL Use

Additional indications for PFCL use include treatment of a rhegmatogenous retinal detachment in which a retinal break cannot be found, subretinal gas, retinal detachments caused by macular holes alone or when a question exists regarding the presence of a second peripheral hole, and submacular hemorrhages.[174]

In a rhegmatogenous retinal detachment without a hole after vitrectomy, PFCL is injected. As the bubble slowly fills the eye, the surgeon looks for schlieren and mixing of the two clear fluids, or unequal density that, when found, marks the site of any retinal tears.[174]

In cases of submacular hemorrhage with a small amount of blood after vitrectomy, the injection of PFCL pushes the subretinal blood anteriorly and out a preexisting retinal hole. With massive subretinal hemorrhage after vitrectomy, subretinal injection of a fibrinolytic agent is made through a retinotomy. On dissolution of the blood clot, intraocular injection of a PFCL pushes the newly liquefied blood out through the retinotomy.[174]

In an eye with a retinal detachment secondary to a macular hole after vitrectomy, injection of a small amount of PFCL flattens the hole and allows laser photocoagulation to be placed around the hole. In the absence of traction on or around the hole, the PFCL does not enter the subretinal space through the hole.[174]

REFERENCES

1. Stone W Jr: Alloplasty in surgery of the eye. *N Engl J Med* 1958;258:486–490.
2. Cibis PA, Becker B, Okun E, et al: The use of liquid silicone in retinal detachment surgery. *Arch Ophthalmol* 1962;68:590–599.
3. Okun E: Intravitreal surgery utilizing liquid silicone: A long term follow-up. *Trans Pac Coast Oto-ophthalmol Soc* 1968;49:141–159.
4. Scott JD: The treatment of massive vitreous retraction by the separation of pre-retinal membranes using liquid silicone. *Mod Probl Ophthalmol* 1975;15:185–190.
5. Leaver PK, Grey RHB, Garner A: Silicone oil injection in the treatment of massive preretinal retraction: II. Late complications in 93 eyes. *Br J Ophthalmol* 1979; 63:361–367.
6. Constable I, Mohamed S, Tan PL: Super viscous silicone liquid in retinal surgery. *Aust J Ophthalmol* 1982;10:5–11.
7. Gonvers M: Temporary use of intraocular silicone oil in the treatment of detachment with massive periretinal proliferation: Preliminary report. *Ophthalmologica* 1982;184:210–218.
8. Živojnović R, Mertens DAE, Peperkamp E: Das flüssige Silikon in der Amotio chirurgie (II): Bericht über 280 Fälle—weitere Entwicklung der Technik. *Klin Monatsbl Augenheilkd* 1982;181:444–452.
9. DeCorral LR, Peyman GA: Pars plana vitrectomy and intravitreal silicone oil injection in eyes with rubeosis iridis. *Can J Ophthalmol* 1986;21:10–12.
10. Peyman GA, Kao GW, de Corral LR: Randomized clinical trial of intraocular silicone vs. gas in the management of complicated retinal detachment and vitreous hemorrhage. *Int Ophthalmol* 1987;10:221–234.
11. Norton EWD, Aaberg T, Fung W, et al: Giant retinal tears: I. Clinical management with intravitreal air. *Am J Ophthalmol* 1969;68:1011–1021.
12. Vygantas CM, Peyman GA, Daily MJ, et al: Octafluorocyclobutane and other gases for vitreous replacement. *Arch Ophthalmol* 1973;90:235–236.
13. Peyman GA, Vygantas CM, Bennett TO, et al: Octafluorocyclobutane in vitreous and aqueous humor replacement. *Arch Ophthalmol* 1975;93:514–517.
14. Lincoff H, Mardirossian J, Lincoff A, et al: Intravitreal longevity of three perfluorocarbon gases. *Arch Ophthalmol* 1980;98:1610–1611.
15. Lincoff H: A small bubble technique for manipulating giant retinal tears. *Ann Ophthalmol* 1981;13:241–243.

16. Lincoff H, Coleman J, Kressig I, et al: The perfluorocarbon gases in the treatment of retinal detachment. *Ophthalmology* 1983;90:546–551.
17. Haut J, Ullern M, Chermet M, et al: Complications of intraocular injections of silicone combined with vitrectomy. *Ophthalmologica* 1980;180:29–35.
18. Meinert H: Requirements of perfluorocarbons for use in ophthalmology. *J Vitreo Retina* 1992;1:5–16.
19. Clark LC Jr, Gollan F: Survival of mammals breathing organic fluids equilibrated with oxygen at atmospheric pressure. *Science* 1966;152:1755–1756.
20. Geyer RP: Fluorocarbon-polyol artificial blood substitutes. *N Engl J Med* 1973; 289:1077–1082.
21. Geyer RP: Oxygen transport in vivo by means of perfluorochemical preparations. *N Engl J Med* 1982;307:304–305.
22. Rude RE, Bush LR, Tilton GD: Effects of fluorocarbons with and without oxygen supplementation on cardiac hemodynamics and energetics. *Am J Cardiol* 1984; 54:880–883.
23. Krucoff MW, Wisdom C, Takeda RN, et al: Quantitative reduction of ischemia during angioplasty: Distal coronary perfusion with oxygenated Fluosol. *Circulation* 1986;74(Suppl II):1446.
24. Jaffe CC, Wohlgelernter D, Cabin H, et al: Preservation of left ventricular ejection fraction during percutaneous transluminal coronary angioplasty by distal transcatheter coronary perfusion of oxygenated Fluosol DA 20%. *Am Heart J* 1988; 115:1156–1164.
25. Birn GP, Blais P: Perfluorocarbon blood substitutes. *Crit Rev Oncol Hematol* 1987;6:311–374.
26. Clark LC Jr: Description, U.S. Patent no. 4,490,351, Dec. 25, 1984.
27. Falco L, Utari S, Esente S: Comparison of different perfluorocarbon liquids. *J Vitreo Retina* 1992;1:17–19.
28. Miyamoto K, Refojo MF, Tolentino FI, et al: Fluorinated oils as experimental vitreous substitutes. *Arch Ophthalmol* 1986;104:1053–1056.
29. Chang S, Reppucci V, Zimmerman NJ, et al: Perfluorocarbon liquids in the management of traumatic retinal detachments. *Ophthalmology* 1989;96:785–792.
30. Pon DM: Chemical characteristics of perfluorocarbon liquids and silicone oil for complex retinal detachments. *Vitreoretinal Surg Technol* 1990;2:6.
31. Chang S: Low viscosity liquid fluorochemicals in vitreous surgery. *Am J Ophthalmol* 1987;103:38–43.
32. Nabih M, Peyman GA, Clark LC Jr, et al: Experimental evaluation of perfluorophenanthrene as a high specific gravity vitreous substitute: A preliminary report. *Ophthalmic Surg* 1989;20:286–293.
33. Blinder KJ, Peyman GA, Paris CL, et al: Vitreon, a new perfluorocarbon. *Br J Ophthalmol* 1991;75:240–244.
34. Paris CL, Peyman GA, Blinder KJ, et al: Surgical technique for managing rhegmatogenous retinal detachment following prosthokeratoplasty. *Retina* 1991; 11:301–304.
35. Peyman GA, Conway MD, Soike KF, et al: Long-term vitreous replacement in primates with intravitreal Vitreon or Vitreon plus silicone. *Ophthalmic Surg* 1991; 22:657–664.
36. Peyman GA, Blinder KJ, Paris CL, et al: Vitreon: A new perfluorocarbon vitreous substitute. *Afro-Asian J Ophthalmol* 1991;10:48–57.

37. Blinder KJ, Peyman GA, Desai UR, et al: Vitreon: A short-term vitreoretinal tamponade. *Br J Ophthalmol* 1992;76:525–528.
38. Schulman JA, Peyman GA, Blinder KJ, et al: Management of giant retinal tears with perfluoroperhydrophenanthrene (Vitreon). *Jpn J Ophthalmol* 1993;37:70–77.
39. Haidt SJ, Clark LC Jr, Ginsberg J: Liquid perfluorocarbon replacement of the eye, abstracted. *Invest Ophthalmol Vis Sci* 1982;22(Suppl):233.
40. Zimmerman NJ, Faris D: The use of N-perfluorocarbon amines in complicated retinal detachments. *Invest Ophthalmol Vis Sci* 1984;25(Suppl):258.
41. Chang S, Zimmerman NJ, Iwamoto T, et al: Experimental vitreous replacement with perfluorotributylamine. *Am J Ophthalmol* 1987;103:29–37.
42. Miyamoto K, Refojo MF, Tolentino FI, et al: Perfluoroether liquid as a long-term vitreous substitute: An experimental study. *Retina* 1984;4:264–268.
43. Long DM, Long DC, Mattrey RF, et al: An overview of perfluoroctylbromide: Application as a synthetic oxygen carrier and imaging agent for X-Ray, ultrasound, and nuclear magnetic resonance. *Biomater Artif Cells Artif Organs* 1988;16 (1–3):411–420.
44. Chang S, Ozmert E, Zimmerman NJ: Intraoperative perfluorocarbon liquids in the management of proliferative vitreoretinopathy. *Am J Ophthalmol* 1988;106: 668–674.
45. Chang S, Lincoff H, Zimmerman NJ, et al: Giant retinal tears: Surgical techniques and results using perfluorocarbon liquids. *Arch Ophthalmol* 1989;107: 761–766.
46. Lavin M: Heavy liquids for postoperative tamponade. *Br J Ophthalmol* 1992; 76:513 514.
47. De Juan E Jr, McCuen B, Tiedeman J: Intraocular tamponade and surface tension. *Surv Ophthalmol* 1985;30:47–51.
48. Sparrow JR, Jayakumar A, Berrocal M, et al: Experimental studies of the combined use of vitreous substitutes of high and low specific gravity. *Retina* 1992; 12:134–140.
49. Velikay M, Wedrich A, Stolba U, et al: Experimental long-term vitreous replacement with purified and nonpurified perfluorodecalin. *Am J Ophthalmol* 1993; 116:565–570.
50. Chang S, Sparrow JR, Iwamoto T, et al: Experimental studies of tolerance to intravitreal perfluoro-n-octane liquid. *Retina* 1991;11:367–374.
51. Sparrow JR, Matthews GP, Iwamoto T, et al: Retinal tolerance to intravitreal perfluoroethylcyclohexane liquid in the rabbit. *Retina* 1993;13:56–62.
52. Eckardt C, Nicolai U, Winter M, et al: Experimental intraocular tolerance to liquid perfluorooctane and perfluoropolyether. *Retina* 1991;11:375–384.
53. Mattrey RF, Scheible FW, Gosink BB, et al: Perfluoroctylbromide: A liver/spleen-specific and tumor-imaging ultrasound contrast material. *Radiology* 1982;145: 759–762.
54. Perk WW, Mattrey RF, Slutsky RA, et al: Perfluoroctylbromide: Acute hemodynamic effects, in pigs, of intravenous administration compared with standard ionic contrast media. *Invest Radiol* 1984;19:129–132.
55. Bruneton JN, Falewée MN, François E, et al: Liver, spleen and vessels: Preliminary clinical results of CT with perfluorooctylbromide. *Radiology* 1989;170:179–183.
56. Flores-Aguilar M, Crapotta JA, Munguia D, et al: Perfluorooctylbromide (PFOB) as a temporary vitreous substitute. *Invest Ophthalmol Vis Sci* 1991; 32(Suppl):1225.
57. Conway MD, Peyman GA, Karaçorlu M, et al: Perfluorooctylbromide (PFOB) as a vitreous substitute in non-human primates. *Int Ophthalmol* 1993;17:259–264.

58. Peyman GA, Blinder KJ, Liu KR, et al: Perfluorophenanthrene: A new vitreous substitute, in Khoo CY, Ang BC, Cheah WM, et al (eds): *New Frontiers in Ophthalmology*. Amsterdam: Elsevier Science Publishers, BV, 1991, pp 605–607.
59. Tanji TM, Peyman GA, Mehta NJ, et al: Perfluoroperhydrophenanthrene (Vitreon) as a short-term vitreous substitute after complex vitreoretinal surgery. *Ophthalmic Surg* 1993;24:681–685.
60. Gremillion CM Jr, Peyman GA, Liu KR, et al: Fluorosilicone oil in the treatment of retinal detachment. *Br J Ophthalmol* 1990;74:643–646.
61. Lobes LA, Burton TC: The incidence of macular pucker after retinal detachment surgery. *Am J Ophthalmol* 1978;83:72–77.
62. McCuen BW, de Juan E Jr, Landers MB, et al: Silicone oil in vitreoretinal surgery: Part 2. Results and complications. *Retina* 1985;5:198–205.
63. Verma LK, Peyman GA, Wafapoor H, et al: An analysis of posterior segment complications after vitrectomy using the perfluorocarbon perfluoroperhydrophenanthrene (Vitreon). (*Ophthalmic Surg*, in press).
64. Greve MDJ, Peyman GA, Millsap CM: Review of the ocular complications and toxicity of liquid perfluorocarbons. *Afro-Asian J Ophthalmol* 1994;12:369–374.
65. Moreira H, de Queiroz JM Jr, Liggett PE, et al: Corneal toxicity study of two perfluorocarbon liquids in rabbit eyes. *Cornea* 1992;11(5):376–379.
66. De Queiroz JM, Blanks JC, Ozler SA, et al: Subretinal perfluorocarbon liquids: An experimental study. *Retina* 1992;12(3 Suppl):S33–S39.
67. Meyer MA, Zak RD: The effect of perfluorophenanthrene liquid on the duration of intraocular perfluorocarbon gas. *Invest Ophthalmol Vis Sci* 1994;35 (Suppl):1617.
68. Stolba U, Krepler K, Pflug R, et al: Experimental vitreous replacement with perfluorophenanthrene: Histological and electrophysiological findings. *Invest Ophthalmol Vis Sci* 1994;35(Suppl):2071.
69. Refojo MF, Araiz J, Arroyo M, et al: The refractive index of Vitreon. *Ophthalmic Surg* 1992;23:436.
70. Peyman GA: Response to Refojo MF, Araiz J, Arroyo M, et al: The refractive index of Vitreon. *Ophthalmic Surg* 1992;23:436.
71. Peyman GA, Mehta NJ: Intravitreal infusion-aspiration instrument for silicone oil–perfluorocarbon liquid exchange. *Retina* 1993;13:177–178.
72. Brown GC, Benson WE: Use of sodium hyaluronate for the repair of giant retinal tears. *Arch Ophthalmol* 1989;107:1246–1249.
73. McDonald HR, Lewis H, Aaberg TM, et al: Complications of endodrainage retinotomies created during vitreous surgery for complicated retinal detachment. *Ophthalmology* 1989;96:358–363.
74. Bottoni F, Bailo G, Arpa P, et al: Management of giant retinal tears using perfluorodecalin as a postoperative short-term vitreoretinal tamponade: A long-term follow-up study. *Ophthalmic Surg* 1994;25:365–373.
75. Joondeph BC, Flynn HW Jr, Blankenship GW, et al: The surgical management of giant retinal tears with the cannulated extrusion needle. *Am J Ophthalmol* 1989; 108:548–553.
76. Haut J, Larricart P, van Effenterre G: Localized retinectomy indications in the treatment and prevention of retinal detachment. *Ophthalmologica* 1984;188: 212–215.
77. Machemer R: Retinotomy. *Am J Ophthalmol* 1981;92:768–774.
78. Ando F, Kondo J: Surgical techniques for giant retinal tears with retinal tacks. *Ophthalmic Surg* 1986;17:408–411.

79. Abrams GW, Williams GA, Neuwirth J, et al: Clinical results of titanium retinal tacks with pneumatic insertion. *Am J Ophthalmol* 1986;102:13–19.
80. Ando F, Kondo J: A plastic tack for the treatment of retinal detachment with giant tear. *Am J Ophthalmol* 1983;95:260–261.
81. De Juan E Jr, McCuen BW II, Machemer R: The use of retinal tacks in the repair of complicated retinal detachments. *Am J Ophthalmol* 1986;102:20–24.
82. O'Grady GE, Parel J-M, Lee W, et al: Hypodermic stainless steel tacks and companion inserter designed for peripheral fixation of retina. *Arch Ophthalmol* 1988; 106:271–275.
83. McCuen BW II, Hida T, Sheta SM: Transvitreal cyanoacrylate retinopexy in the management of complicated retinal detachment. *Am J Ophthalmol* 1987;104: 127–132.
84. Millsap CM, Peyman GA, Mehta NJ, et al: Vitreon in the management of giant retinal tears: Results of a collaborative study. *Ophthalmic Surg* 1993;24:759–763.
85. Glaser BM, Carter JB, Kuppermann BD, et al: Perfluoro-octane in the treatment of giant retinal tears with proliferative vitreoretinopathy. *Ophthalmology* 1991;98: 1613–1621.
86. Kreiger AE, Lewis H: Management of giant retinal tears without scleral buckling: Use of radical dissection of the vitreous base and perfluoro-octane and intraocular tamponade. *Ophthalmology* 1992;99:491–497.
87. Le Mer Y, Kroll P: Liquid perfluorocarbon in treatment of giant tears. *Klin Monatsbl Augenheilkd* 1991;199(4):256–258.
88. Forlini C: Centrifugal surgical strategy with early introduction of PFCL in the management of retinal tractional detachment: Effect on reproliferation. *J Vitreo Retina* 1992;1:44–51.
89. Carroll BF, Peyman GA, Mehta NJ: Repair of retinal detachment associated with proliferative vitreoretinopathy using perfluoroperhydrophenanthrene (Vitreon). *Can J Ophthalmol* 1994;29:66–69.
90. Peyman GA, Schulman JA: *Intravitreal Surgery: Principles and Practice.* Norwalk, CT: Appleton & Lange, 1994, pp 620–621.
91. Liu K-R, Peyman GA, Chen M-S, et al: Use of high-density vitreous substitutes in the removal of posteriorly dislocated lenses or intraocular lenses. *Ophthalmic Surg* 1991;22:503–507.
92. Greve MDJ, Peyman GA, Mehta NJ, et al: Use of perfluoroperhydrophenanthrene in the management of posteriorly dislocated crystalline and intraocular lenses. *Ophthalmic Surg* 1993;24:593–597.
93. Korobelnik JF, Nabet L, Frau E, et al: Utilisation des perfluorocarbones liquides dans le traitement chirurgical des luxations posterieures du cristallin. *J Fr Ophtalmol* 1992:15:235–242.
94. Shapiro MJ, Resnick KI, Kim SH, et al: Management of the dislocated crystalline lens with a perfluorocarbon liquid. *Am J Ophthalmol* 1991;112:401–405.
95. Van Effenterre G, Le Mer Y, Lacotte JL, et al: Luxation posterieure du cristallin ou d'un implant: Traitement chirurgical utilisant un perfluorocarbone liquid. *J Fr Ophtalmol* 1992;13:337.
96. Rowson NJ, Bacon AS, Rosen PH: Perfluorocarbon heavy liquids in the management of posterior dislocation of the lens nucleus during phakoemulsification. *Br J Ophthalmol* 1992;76:169–170.
97. Le Mer Y, Haut J, Van Effenterre G, et al: Use of perfluorocarbon liquid in the management of posterior dislocation of the lens. *J Vitreo Retina* 1992;1:53–54.

98. Wallace RT, McNamara JA, Brown G, et al: The use of perfluorophenanthrene in the removal of intravitreal lens fragments. *Am J Ophthalmol* 1993;116:196–200.
99. Lewis H, Sanchez G: The use of perfluorocarbon liquids in the repositioning of posteriorly dislocated intraocular lenses. *Ophthalmology* 1993;100:1055–1059.
100. Ong SG, Heng LK, Tan BB, et al: Perfluorocarbon liquids (perfluorodecalin) in vitreoretinal surgery: A local experience. *Annals of the Academy of Medicine, Singapore* 1993;22(3):348–350.
101. Fanous MM, Friedman SM: Ciliary sulcus fixation of a dislocated posterior chamber intraocular lens using liquid perfluorophenanthrene. *Ophthalmic Surg* 1992; 23:551–552.
102. Lewis H, Blumenkranz MS, Chang S: Treatment of dislocated crystalline lens and retinal detachment with perfluorocarbon liquids. *Retina* 1992;12:299–304.
103. Brod RD, Flynn HW Jr, Clarkson JG, et al: Management options for retinal detachment in the presence of a posteriorly dislocated intraocular lens. *Retina* 1990; 10:50–56.
104. Lakhanpal V, Schocket SS, Elman MJ, et al: Intraoperative massive suprachoroidal hemorrhage during pars plana vitrectomy. *Ophthalmology* 1990;97: 1114–1119.
105. Whitehouse GM, Filipic M, Francis IC: Expulsive choroidal haemorrhage: A clinical and pathological review. *Aust N Z J Ophthalmol* 1989;17(3):225–232.
106. Chu TG, Cano MR, Green RL, et al: Massive suprachoroidal hemorrhage with central retinal apposition: A clinical and echographic study. *Arch Ophthalmol* 1991; 109:1575–1581.
107. Givens K, Shields MB: Suprachoroidal hemorrhage after glaucoma filtering surgery. *Am J Ophthalmol* 1987;103:689–694.
108. Luntz MH, Rosenblatt M: Malignant glaucoma: Major review. *Surv Ophthalmol* 1987;32:73–93.
109. Jaffe NS: *Cataract Surgery and Its Complications*, 4th ed. St. Louis: CV Mosby, 1984, pp 489–496.
110. Bukelman A, Hoffman P, Oliver M: Limited choroidal hemorrhage associated with extracapsular cataract extraction. *Arch Ophthalmol* 1987;105:338–341.
111. Davison JA: Acute intraoperative suprachoroidal hemorrhage in extracapsular cataract surgery. *J Cataract Refract Surg* 1986;12:606–622.
112. Payne JW, Kameen AJ, Jensen AD, et al: Expulsive hemorrhage: Its incidence in cataract surgery and a report of four bilateral cases. *Trans Am Ophthalmol Soc* 1985;83:181–204.
113. Machemer R, Laqua H: A logical approach to the treatment of massive periretinal proliferation. *Ophthalmology* 1978;85:584–593.
114. Hawkins WR, Schepens CL: Choroidal detachment and retinal surgery: A clinical and experimental study. *Am J Ophthalmol* 1966;62:813–819.
115. Wolter JR: Expulsive hemorrhage during retinal detachment surgery: A case with survival of the eye after Verhoeff sclerotomy. *Am J Ophthalmol* 1961;51:264–266.
116. Bellows AR, Chylack LT Jr, Hutchinson BT: Choroidal detachment: Clinical manifestation, therapy, and mechanism of formation. *Ophthalmology* 1981;88: 1107–1115.
117. Manschot WA: The pathology of expulsive hemorrhage. *Am J Ophthalmol* 1955; 40:15–24.
118. Maumenee AE, Schwartz MF: Acute intraoperative choroidal effusion. *Am J Ophthalmol* 1985;100:147–154.

198   VITREOUS SUBSTITUTES

119. Zauberman H: Expulsive choroidal haemorrhage: An experimental study. *Br J Ophthalmol* 1982;66:43–45.
120. Beyer CF, Peyman GA, Hill JM: Expulsive choroidal hemorrhage in rabbits: A histopathologic study. *Arch Ophthalmol* 1989;107:1648–1653.
121. Freeman WR, Schneiderman TE, Weinreb RN, et al: Hemorrhagic choroidal detachment with anterior vitreoretinal adhesions. *Ophthalmic Surg* 1991;22: 670–675.
122. Welch JC, Spaeth GL, Benson WE: Massive suprachoroidal hemorrhage: Follow-up and outcome of 30 cases. *Ophthalmology* 1988;95:1202–1206.
123. Purcell JJ Jr, Krachmer JH, Doughman DJ, et al: Expulsive hemorrhage in penetrating keratoplasty. *Ophthalmology* 1982;89:41–43.
124. Frenkel REP, Shin DH: Prevention and management of delayed suprachoroidal hemorrhage after filtration surgery. *Arch Ophthalmol* 1986;104: 1459–1463.
125. Speaker MG, Guerriero PN, Met JA, et al: A case-control study of risk factors for intraoperative suprachoroidal expulsive hemorrhage. *Ophthalmology* 1991;98: 202–210.
126. Hoffman P, Pollack A, Oliver M: Limited choroidal hemorrhage associated with intracapsular cataract extraction. *Arch Ophthalmol* 1984;102:1761–1765.
127. Gressel MG, Parrish RK II, Heuer DK: Delayed nonexpulsive suprachoroidal hemorrhage. *Arch Ophthalmol* 1984;102:1757–1760.
128. Simmons RJ: Filtering operations, in Epstein DL (ed): *Chandler and Grant's Glaucoma*, 3rd ed. Philadelphia: Lea & Febiger, 1986, pp 444–446.
129. Abrams GW, Thomas MA, Williams GA, et al: Management of postoperative suprachoroidal hemorrhage with continuous-infusion air pump. *Arch Ophthalmol* 1986;104:1455–1458.
130. Lakhanpal V, Schocket SS, Elman MJ, et al: A new modified vitreoretinal surgical approach in the management of massive suprachoroidal hemorrhage. *Ophthalmology* 1989;96:793–800.
131. Baldwin LB, Smith TJ, Hollins JL, et al: The use of viscoelastic substances in the drainage of postoperative suprachoroidal hemorrhage. *Ophthalmic Surg* 1989; 20:504–507.
132. Peyman GA, Mafee M, Schulman J: Computed tomography in choroidal detachment. *Ophthalmology* 1984;91:156–162.
133. Coleman DJ, Wilcox LM Jr: The choroid: Its function, evaluation, and surgical management, in *Symposium on Medical and Surgical Diseases of the Retina and Vitreous: Transactions of the New Orleans Academy of Ophthalmology*. St Louis: CV Mosby, 1983, pp 1–24.
134. Byer NE: The natural history of senile retinoschisis. *Trans Am Acad Ophthalmol Otolaryngol* 1976;81:458–471.
135. Peyman GA, Carney MD: Combined internal drainage of subretinal fluid and choroidal detachment. *Int Ophthalmol* 1987;10:41–46.
136. Desai UR, Peyman GA, Chen CJ, et al: The use of perfluoroperhydrophenanthrene in the management of suprachoroidal hemorrhages. *Ophthalmology* 1992;99: 1542–1547.
137. Ruderman JM, Harbin TS Jr, Campbell DG: Postoperative suprachoroidal hemorrhage following filtration procedures. *Arch Ophthalmol* 1986;104:201–205.
138. Davison JA: Vitrectomy and fluid infusion in the treatment of delayed suprachoroidal hemorrhage after combined cataract and glaucoma filtration surgery. *Ophthalmic Surg* 1987;18:334–336.

139. Dannemann AF, Majerovics A, Kaback MB: Documentation of suprachoroidal hemorrhage during B-scan ultrasonography. *Arch Ophthalmol* 1989;107:960.

140. Desai UR, Peyman GA, Harper CA, et al: The use of Vitreon in the removal of massive vitreous hemorrhage caused by perforating ocular trauma. *Invest Ophthalmol Vis Sci* 1992;33(Suppl):1314.

141. Spencer WH: *Ophthalmic Pathology: An Atlas and Textbook*, 3rd ed, vol. 3. Philadelphia: WB Saunders, 1986, pp 1415–1424.

142. Hanneken A, de Juan E Jr, McCuen BW II: The management of retinal detachments associated with choroidal colobomas by vitreous surgery. *Am J Ophthalmol* 1991;111:271–275.

143. McDonald HR, Lewis H, Brown G, et al: Vitreous surgery for retinal detachment associated with choroidal coloboma. *Arch Ophthalmol* 1991;109:1399–1402.

144. Jesberg DO, Schepens CL: Retinal detachment associated with coloboma of the choroid. *Arch Ophthalmol* 1961;65:163–173.

145. Patnaik B, Kalsi R: Retinal detachment with coloboma of the choroid. *Ind J Ophthalmol* 1981;29:345–349.

146. Schepens CL: *Retinal Detachment and Allied Diseases*, vol. 2. Philadelphia: WB Saunders, 1983, pp 615–617.

147. Dufour R: Survey of statistics on juvenile detachment. *Mod Probl Ophthalmol* 1969;8:358–362.

148. Zhang FK: Congenital coloboma of the choroid with retinal detachment. *Tianjin J Med* 1978;4:173–178.

149. Wang K, Hilton GF: Retinal detachment associated with coloboma of the choroid. *Trans Am Ophthalmol Soc* 1985;83:49.

150. Bao LL: Retinal detachment associated with congenital coloboma of the choroid. *Chung-Hua Yen Ko Tsa Chih* 1980;16:165–169.

151. Gonvers M: Temporary use of silicone oil in the treatment of special cases of retinal detachment. *Ophthalmologica* 1983;187:202–209.

152. Gopal L, Kini MM, Badrinath SS, et al: Management of retinal detachment with choroidal coloboma. *Ophthalmology* 1991;98:1622–1627.

153. Michels RG, Wilkinson CP, Rice TA: *Retinal Detachment*. St. Louis: CV Mosby, 1990, pp 727–730.

154. Lee KJ, Peyman GA, Paris CL, et al: Management of retinal detachment associated with choroidal coloboma using perfluoroperhydrophenanthrene (Vitreon). *Ophthalmic Surg* 1992;23:553–554.

155. Barron BA: Prosthokeratoplasty, in Kaufman HE, Barron BA, McDonald MB, et al (eds): *The Cornea*. New York: Churchill Livingstone, 1988, pp 787–803.

156. Cardona H: Prosthokeratoplasty. *Cornea* 1983;2:179–183.

157. Buxton J, Norden RA: Adult penetrating keratoplasty: Indications and contraindications, in Brightbill FS (ed): *Corneal Surgery: Theory, Technique and Tissue*. St. Louis: CV Mosby, 1986, pp 129–140.

158. Barron BA, Dingeldein S, Kaufman HE: Spontaneous unscrewing of a Cardona keratoprosthesis. *Am J Ophthalmol* 1987;103:331–332.

159. Girard LJ: Keratoprosthesis. *Cornea* 1983;2:207–224.

160. Barber JC: Keratoprosthesis: Past and present. *Int Ophthalmol Clin* 1988;28:103–109.

161. Aquavella JV, Rao GN, Brown AC, et al: Keratoprosthesis: Results, complications, and management. *Ophthalmology* 1982;89:655–660.

162. Rao GN, Blatt HL, Aquavella JV: Results of keratoprosthesis. *Am J Ophthalmol* 1979;88:190–204.

163. Maguire AM, Trese MT: Lens-sparing vitreoretinal surgery in infants. *Arch Ophthalmol* 1992;110:284–286.
164. Lambert HM, Capone A Jr, Aaberg TM, et al: Surgical excision of subfoveal neovascular membranes in age-related macular degeneration. *Am J Ophthalmol* 1992;113:257–262.
165. Corcostegui B: Use of perfluorocarbon liquid in vitrectomy for diabetic rhegmatogenous retinal detachment. *J Vitreo Retina* 1992;1:30–34.
166. Mathis A: The use of perfluorodecalin in diabetic vitrectomy. *J Vitreo Retina* 1992;1:28–29.
167. Forlini C, Dal Fiume E, Cicognani A, et al: Use of PFCL in the surgical management of endophthalmitis: New indication. *J Vitreo Retina* 1992;1:55–63.
168. Peyman GA, Alturki WA, Nelson NC Jr: Surgical management of incarcerated retina in the sclerotomy. *Ophthalmic Surg* 1992;23:628–629.
169. Skolik SA, Moreira CA, Freeman WR, et al: Liquid perfluorocarbons for control of bleeding during pars plana vitrectomy: An animal model and human clinical correlation. *Invest Ophthalmol Vis Sci* 1994;35(Suppl):1618.
170. Resnick KI, Shapiro MJ, Kim S: Perfluorooctane as an instrument to manipulate intraocular foreign bodies. *Invest Ophthalmol Vis Sci* 1991;32(Suppl):881.
171. Sargent JW, Seffl RJ: Properties of perfluorinated liquids. *Fed Proc* 1970;29:1699–1703.
172. Berkowitz BA, Wilson CA, Hatchell DL: Oxygen kinetics in the vitreous substitute perfluorotributylamine: A ^{19}F NMR study in vivo. *Invest Ophthalmol Vis Sci* 1991;32:2382–2397.
173. Wilson CA, Berkowitz BA, Srebro R: Perfluorinated vitreous substitute increased retinal tolerance to ischemia. *Invest Ophthalmol Vis Sci* 1994; 35(Suppl):2070.
174. Berrocal MH, Chang S: Perfluorocarbon liquids in vitreous surgery. *Ophthalmology Clin North Am* 1994;7(1):67–76.

Index

Note: Page numbers in italics refer to figures and tables.

recurrence of, 4, 10–11, 18–20, *19,* 32, 39
  and silicone oil, 38
  traumatic type of, 38, 175, *176,* 177–180
  treatments for, 3–5, 18, 22, 37, 53, 77,
    78–80, 80, 148
  See also retinal tears; rhegmatogenous
    retinal detachments; tamponades
retinal folds
  complications with, 119
  elimination of, 53, 98
  manual unfolding of, 155
  posterior, 75
  xenon for, 70
retinal holes, 42, 77, 85
retinal perforator, 85
retinal tacks, 156
retinal tears
  causes of, 103–104
  iatrogenic, 42
  inferior type of, 2
  localization of, *81–83*
  and PFCLs, 175, *176,* 177–180
  pneumatic retinopexy for, 97–98
  and preparation for injections, 4
  reopening of, 106
  See also giant retinal tears; retinal
    detachments; tamponades
retinoic acid, 40
retinol, 6, 40
retinopathy of prematurity (ROP), 183–184,
    184, 185, 186
retinopexy, 74, 178–179. *See also*
  pneumatic retinopexy
retinotomy
  complications in, 87
  and drainage, 80, 85
  frequency of, 38
  indications for, 42, 156
  and membrane epicenters, 41
  sites for, 84–85
  and subretinal air, 109, *110*
  for subretinal silicone oil, *30*
retrobulbar anesthesia, 90, 93, 99
retrocorneal membrane, *12, 13*
retrohyaloid space, 106, 177
retrolental space, 107
rhegmatogenous retinal detachments
  and air or gas injection, 53, 121
  PFCLs used for, 151, *153,* 191

pneumatic retinopexy for, 107–109
prosthokeratoplasty for, 180–183, *181*
and retinal folds, 75
scleral buckling for, 104, 107–109
treatments for, 18, 97
Riedel KG, 35
Ringer's solution, 138, 167
Rinkoff JS, 41, 42
Rosengren B, 53
rubeosis, 16, 39–41

S

Sabates WI, 59
scatter laser photocoagulation, 43
Schenk H, 54
Schiotz tonometry, 72–73
schlieren, 177–178
Schubert HD, 11, 16, 22, 32
scleral buckling
  and air–fluid exchanges, *88*
  for choroidal coloboma, 177–178
  complications with, 120
  and gas injection, 70, 75
  for giant retinal tears, 119–121
  indications for, 2, 24, 156, 187
  for phakic eyes, 107–108
  and pneumatic retinopexy, 98, 103,
    107–109
  for retinopathy of prematurity, 186
  success rates for, 103
  techniques for using, 31
Scott JD, 6, 32
Sebag J, 104
segmentation, 119
Sell CH, 32
serum, 9
Setälä K, 12
SF_6. *See* sulfur hexafluoride gas (SF_6)
Shields CL, 5
Shin DH, 170
shunt implants, 18
Si-C bonds, 14
silica, 15
silicone–air exchanges, 156
silicone–fluid exchange, 27, 32
silicone oil keratopathy
  development of, 12–15